MANAGING
HEALTH CARE

The Management of Health Care

Series Editors
John J. Glynn & David A. Perkins

Other titles in the series:

The Clinician's Management Handbook

Managing Health Service Contracts

Achieving Value for Money

The GP's Management Handbook

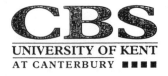

CBS
UNIVERSITY OF KENT
AT CANTERBURY ■■■■

MANAGING HEALTH CARE

Challenges for the 90s

Edited by

John J. Glynn

and

David A. Perkins

Canterbury Business School, University of Kent

WB Saunders Company Ltd

London   Philadelphia   Toronto   Sydney   Tokyo

W. B. Saunders Company Ltd   24–28 Oval Road
London NW1 7DX

The Curtis Center
Independence Square West
Philadelphia, PA 19106–3399, USA

Harcourt Brace & Company
55 Horner Avenue
Toronto, Ontario M8Z 4X6, Canada

Harcourt Brace & Company, Australia
30–52 Smidmore Street
Marrickville, NSW 2204, Australia

Harcourt Brace & Company, Japan
Ichibancho Central Building, 22–1 Ichibancho
Chiyoda-ku, Tokyo 102, Japan

A catalogue record of this book is available from the British Library

ISBN 0-7020-1831-7

Typeset by Paston Press Ltd, Loddon, Norfolk
Printed and bound in Great Britain by WBC, Bridgend, Mid Glamorgan

CONTENTS

CONTRIBUTORS

Alison Baker   Management Development Manager, Institute of Health Services Management, London.

Louise Bell   Medical Audit Co-ordinator, Southend Health Care NHS Trust, Essex.

Michael Calnan   Professor of Sociology of Health Studies, and Director of the Centre for Health Services Studies, University of Kent at Canterbury.

Malcolm Forsythe   Professorial Fellow in Public Health, Centre for Health Services Studies, University of Kent at Canterbury.

John J. Glynn   Professor of Financial Management and founding Director of Canterbury Business School, University of Kent at Canterbury.

Andrew Gray   Reader in Public Accountability and Management, Canterbury Business School, University of Kent at Canterbury.

David J. Hunter   Professor of Health Policy and Management, and Director, Nuffield Institute for Health, University of Leeds.

William I. Jenkins   Reader in Public Policy and Management, Darwin College, University of Kent at Canterbury.

Martin Knapp   Professor of the Economics of Social Care, Personal Social Sciences Research Unit, University of Kent at Canterbury and Professor and Director of the Centre for the Economics of Mental Health, Institute of Psychiatry, University of London.

Robyn Lawson   Training and Development Officer, North Kent Healthcare NHS Trust, Sittingbourne.

Barbara Morris   Senior Lecturer in Operations Management, Canterbury Business School, University of Kent at Canterbury.

David A. Perkins   Lecturer in Strategic Management and Director of MBA, Canterbury Business School, University of Kent at Canterbury.

Carl R. Whitehouse   Professor of Teaching Medicine in the Community, Department of General Practice, University of Manchester.

ACKNOWLEDGEMENTS

The cartoons which appear on the section openings are reproduced by kind permission of the following:

Michael Cummings, *Daily Express*, 27 March 1950, Syndication Department, Express Newspapers plc, London.

David Low, *Evening Standard*, 19 May 1944, Solo Syndication and Literary Agency, London.

Emmwood (John Musgrave-Wood), *Sunday Dispatch*, 24 April 1960, Solo Syndication and Literary Agency, London.

John Jensen, *Sunday Telegraph*, 7 June 1970, Ewan MacNaughton Associates, Tonbridge, Kent.

All the cartoons were obtained with the kind assistance of the Centre for the Study of Cartoons and Caricature, University of Kent, Canterbury, UK.

We would also like to acknowledge the Office of Health Economics, 12 Whitehall, London, UK, for permission to reproduce extracts from their *Compendium of Health Statistics*, 7th edition, 1992, which appear in Chapter 8, *Acute Services*.

FOREWORD

Professor Karol Sikora

The only constancy in Britain's NHS today seems to be change. As we approach the fiftieth anniversary of this remarkable institution, many clinicians are full of gloom and despondency. Some complain that they just do not understand what went wrong. The truth of course is that times have changed for all the professions whether in medicine, education, the civil service or government. They are not the cosy, unaccountable, highly respected and well paid jobs that our predecessors seemed to have. In fact nothing has gone wrong – some just find adapting to the new culture more difficult than others.

This short, compelling and very readable book provides a remarkable insight into the way in which healthcare is being managed and changed in Britain. The demand for technologically driven, highly specialized medicine is insatiable. Rationing is an implicit part of management. Who better to do this than doctors, who can really grasp the disadvantages as well as benefits, often through a confused web of hype created by powerful vested interests. Direct accountability for resources and ensuring quality are now an implicit role for those involved in service management. Clinical directors are ideally placed to take on this task even though colleagues may find the potential erosion of their clinical freedom unwelcome.

This volume provides an excellent introduction to the external and internal forces operating on healthcare provision. Society and its expectations have changed. Waiting four hours for a five minute consultation with the great man is just no longer good enough. The rise of consumerism in medicine is inexorable and is driven in part by the political process. Value for money, greater accountability, competition and consumer responsiveness are essential components throughout the public sector. Here you will see how the NHS Management Executive produces an overall strategy. This is followed by the management of the most important part of the service – its staff. With over one million workers, by far the biggest UK employer, it is quite amazing how low its human resources are valued.

You will find information on the management of quality, purchasing choices, community services, general practice, changing patterns of care and consumerism. The inevitable conflicts of the new marketplace, the realignment of old loyalties and the changing ways in which health care is provided have left some serious casualties in the form of closed hospitals and once powerful institutions whose influence is now declining.

The pace of change is relentless and will continue to be so. The post war baby boom is going to create a huge increase in the elderly within 25 years. And medical advances driven by a strange mixture of altruism, curiosity, ambition and profit will make what is impossible today the routine of tomorrow.

Every doctor, and as you will see there are nearly 60 000 of us, should read this book as its contents will profoundly affect their every working day whatever their specialty. We are all in it together facing up to the contradiction of trying to get more out of less. Chief executives should buy it for every Clinical Director. No healthcare manager can afford not to thoroughly understand its contents.

John Glynn and David Perkins are to be congratulated for putting together such a superb guide to this highly complex field. It is a unique contribution which will help us all shape the way forward for the NHS.

Karol Sikora

Professor of Clinical Oncology, Royal Postgraduate Medical School and Joint Director for Cancer Services, Hammersmith and Charing Cross Hospitals.

INTRODUCTION

John J. Glynn and David A. Perkins

SETTING THE SCENE

To say to clinicians or anyone else involved in the provision of health care that we live in interesting times would be scoffed at as the understatement of the decade. If we confine ourselves to the recent history of the National Health Service (NHS) we can see fundamental reforms in both the approach to patient care and the overall management of the service. No longer do we talk about administration of the service, instead we talk of the **management of health care**. The notion of a single unified service has gone and is unlikely to be resurrected. We are, like it or not, in the age of markets, including the market for health care. In the case of the NHS we use the term 'internal market' as though it were some cosy division of responsibilities. In fact nothing could be further from the truth.

- Firstly, the so-called internal market is nothing of the sort since purchasers can buy from private sector providers and some NHS provider facilities are now being slowly privatized themselves.
- Secondly, a market usually denotes buyers and sellers who negotiate on price and quality of service. The problem is that in this market cost is supposed to equal price. Through close regulation of the costing procedures and processes the Secretary of State effectively determines price.
- Thirdly, the market has created several uncertainties about the overall direction of health care. Who is the protector of patient rights? Will any overall strategy for health care research be maintained? What are the career opportunities for clinicians and other professionals in the 1990s?

Peter Griffiths, former Deputy Chief Executive of the NHS Management Executive and a key player in instituting the market philosophy into health care, has recently offered the view that in the longer term the government will purchase health from a completely privatized NHS (*Health Services Journal* 1994). Although this seems unlikely it is fairly clear that many elements of the reforms introduced in recent years will not disappear whatever the political party in power.

Clinicians have always been and still are key stakeholders in the NHS. Until the 1990s NHS administrative changes largely bypassed them or resulted in participative and consultative procedures which uniquely provided them with a collective veto. It was usually the case that until doctors reached the status of Senior Registrar or Consultant in the hospital or worked in the community as a general practitioner (GP), they usually had little or no idea about management issues. They performed their medical duties whilst others organized the institutional and support services for themselves and their patients. Management issues were largely ignored in their years of training but they were always appraised that there were never sufficient resources and that this was not their problem but somebody else's. For those outside the NHS it is incredible to think that clinicians were, and in many instances still are, so marginalized in the management of the NHS.

It might be interesting to analyse some of the historical reasons why this situation arose; however we leave that to others (Watkin 1978; Mackenzie 1979; Klein 1992). The concern of the editors and those who contributed to this book was to create a much greater awareness in clinicians and other health care professionals of the management problems of the late 1990s. Why does this warrant treatment in such depth? The authors believe it is now clear that anyone aspiring to senior positions within this reformed NHS can only do so if they are prepared to take on managerial responsibilities that require their direct accountability for the resources they use and the overall quality of care they provide.

It is no longer feasible for clinicians to ignore the economic consequences of the patient care they provide. Many will say that working in such an environment is not what they expected when they entered training many years ago. That may be true but the very nature of the market cannot even pretend towards efficiency if clinicians are not directly contributing in a number of very positive ways.

♦ Who else can determine the respective protocols for patient care?
♦ Who else can best market the services on offer or determine the particular specifications of a purchaser contract?
♦ Finally one might also ask, who else can defend the development of clinical practice if not the clinicians themselves?

Whether we like it or not there has arisen a view over recent years that the NHS has lacked true public scrutiny, that the NHS has wasted millions of pounds that could have been redirected to more patient care, that bad management practices have led to unnecessary queueing for treatment, that clinicians have been far too slow to adapt to take advantage of the opportunities offered by day surgery and community care (Butler 1992). The hospital consultant was a person who was never challenged. Junior doctors suffered in silence at their treatment. GPs felt marginalized once their patient transferred to a hospital clinic.

These views are not just those of the Conservative government. If they were so they might be easier to ignore. These complaints have been voiced generally in the media, by GPs, and by patients themselves. The concern perhaps is that because *all* those involved in the NHS, from successive Secretaries of State to the hospital ward orderly, have never really faced up to this looming crisis; the changes when they came were far more radical than might really have been necessary and have come at a pace and price that is difficult to comprehend.

As such, therefore, this is a politically neutral book. It does not offer a socio-political critique of the NHS as a national institution. This is a pragmatic book which examines the current NHS environment and the ways in which clinicians are adapting to new requirements. Our aim is to assist clinicians to become much better informed about a whole series of management issues. By doing so we hope that clinicians will be better able to make an effective contribution when it comes to addressing many of the operational and strategic dilemmas faced within the NHS.

WHAT ARE THE MANAGEMENT CHALLENGES?

With this, perhaps contentious, introduction we briefly review the various contributions to this volume. Each chapter stands alone, but we believe they address collectively the key management issues of the 1990s. Each chapter necessarily deals with various issues from slightly different perspectives. Obvious examples include contract management, quality of care and inter-agency relationships. Further volumes in this series will build upon the core themes introduced here. They will discuss in much more detail specific issues, including contracting and value-for-money, and will consider management issues relating to a particular clinical interest group.

We do not offer a simple recipe for successful management of clinical services in the NHS. It is too soon to create a definitive map of the landscape, because the major features are fluid and have not yet taken on a recognizable and consistent form. It is not clear how many GPs will want to manage practice funds or if some of the 'super-fundholders' will be successful. The authors have been selected for their personal experiences and insights. These have not been compressed or recycled into a homogeneous picture; rather the authors have been allowed to describe those aspects of the picture which they are well positioned to observe and the differences of view mirror important contradictions with which clinicians, managers, and patients have to deal.

Neither is it appropriate to wait for the picture to become clearer as it never does. Things do not settle down since the competing demands made of public services, and health services in particular, highlight the structure of interests in our society. Health is only a top priority when it is threatened or when the quality of life is reduced by disease or injury. It follows that health services must compete for attention with a wide range of other interests and its protagonists are seldom content with the resources which they are able to obtain. For instance, the social security budget is approximately twice the size of the health budget although funds are often spent on related problems.

We have divided the book into four sections:

◆ Section I attempts to map the major political developments that have moulded the current political and governmental context.
◆ Section II describes the services from the complementary perspectives of strategy, finance, staffing and quality.
◆ Section III addresses the particular service contexts of primary care, community and acute services, ending with a review of the patient's perspective as consumer.
◆ Section IV concludes by highlighting those major themes of the book that we believe will constitute a critical agenda for the health services, and particularly for the senior clinician who endeavours to combine medical and managerial roles.

I: The impact of government

While the most obvious development to influence health care in recent years might appear to be the creation and introduction of the internal market, such a bald analysis would be simplistic in the extreme. In Chapter 1, **Andrew Gray** and **Bill Jenkins** detail the impact of the political process in the last two decades, highlighting the important processes which have been set in motion and which form the landscape for our review. They place the impact of Thatcherism in a wider context in which governments were seeking greater accountability from public services together with major improvements in value-for-money.

II: Perspectives on NHS management

This section assesses a variety of attempts to shape today's health services. These approaches are not discrete but each has its champions and they have all resulted in the introduction of new management approaches and frameworks within the service.

In Chapter 2, **David Hunter** takes on the herculean task of examining strategy-making in the NHS. How have the various stakeholders attempted to fashion the structure of the service, adjust its direction, and most importantly improve its performance? Even during the periods when there were real annual increases in the resources available to the NHS there was no consistently successful system by which the service could be directed. Periods of resource constraint made the management of the service increasingly disjointed. From the literature he makes it clear that neither private nor public enterprises are clear about what constitutes an effective strategic process. At all levels, clinicians and their representatives, politicians and managers have attempted to change the pattern of services to achieve best value for taxpayer and patient. Dealing with problems like AIDS and cancer would seem to require a strategy – yet do we know how the direction and performance of publicly funded health services can be influenced for the better?

The proper use of limited finance might be seen as one of the key drivers of attempts to reform the management and provision of health services. In Chapter 3, **John Glynn** looks at the way in which new financial systems have been introduced to answer many of the criticisms faced by the service. The failure to be able to locate proper personal accountability for public resources, linked with the common criticism that NHS clinicians and managers did not know what any service, procedure or item of equipment cost, meant that decisions were often taken in ignorance and that critical questions of efficiency and value-for-money were unanswerable. He describes the new financial arrangements which have been progressively introduced, culminating with the financial regime and arrangements of the market.

Most of the money which has to be managed is spent on staff in clinical and support roles. In a real sense the pattern of service stems from the pattern of staffing in the NHS. In Chapter 4, **Alison Baker** and **David Perkins** look at the management of what is increasingly referred to as the human resource. While for many it is hard to find a less pleasant piece of jargon, the provision of high-quality and efficient services does require high standards of staff management by service managers. To ensure that the right people with the right skills are available when needed, without wasting money on unnecessary training or overmanning, is a true skill and requires planning and management at all levels of the NHS.

In Chapter 5, the final contribution in this section, **Barbara Morris** and **Louise Bell** write about quality. Clinicians have had better grounds than most for trusting in the quality of their work and they have had more mechanisms and procedures than most for quality assurance. Unfortunately the service experienced by a patient or a community is a combination of the plans, activities, and actions of a wide range of individuals, teams and organizations. In the past it might have been acceptable for clinicians to call on professional judgement as an arbiter of appropriate quality. Things have changed. Now each of the stakeholders in health care has a view of quality and there has arisen a plethora of experts to identify what systems make for good quality. The market demands a contract of quality, price and volume, and while hard-pressed purchasers might focus on the latter two, high-cost providers will be very keen to demonstrate the superior quality of their services.

III: Managing key services   Good-quality health care may take place in a variety of settings, be provided by a variety of agents, and require a complex pattern of coordination and timing. Clarity of discussion, and the limitations of individual experience, demands that we look at the range of services and their management in parts – but we should not forget that the key to good-quality services is interdependence and cooperation.

Carl Whitehouse writes as a practising GP in Chapter 6, and starts from the position that every individual requires a primary care service that will respond promptly to his or her particular needs. From this starting point in primary care begins a chain of relationships with other providers which GPs have to manage effectively. The market mechanism and the introduction of fund-holding have changed the pattern of services, introducing new possibilities and complexities for GPs and for other providers. The decisions of GPs are increasingly influencing the configuration of community and acute services which form the subject of the following two chapters.

Two key phenomena with which the NHS has to deal are the ageing of the UK population and the changes in technology of medicine. Chapter 7, by **Martin Knapp** and **Robyn Lawson**, shows how developments in community services have attempted to keep pace with an ageing population. They provide an introduction to the complexities of the community care sector, placing particular emphasis on its relationship to the NHS and showing how new patterns of planning, administration and finance have enabled joint programmes of care.

In Chapter 8, **Malcolm Forsythe** looks at advances in acute hospital services which follow from improvements in medical technology and new ideas about what constitute appropriate and effective patterns of care. He shows how public and professional expectations of the acute hospital have developed and points to the impact of major findings about the effectiveness of specialist medical services.

The last chapter in this section, Chapter 9, adopts the patient's perspective as consumer. **Michael Calnan** shows us how expectations have changed – from the widespread assumption of an obedient patient who follows the instructions of the professional, to patients who expect to be consulted about the pattern of their treatment. He describes how the development of consumerism in the wider society has influenced government policies and become a matter of daily concern in each part of the NHS. Clinicians in managerial positions can no longer afford to neglect the issue of consumer influence, nor can their colleagues hide under the mantle of patient management or clinical judgement.

IV: The management agenda for senior clinicians

In the final section, Chapter 10 highlights some of the most important common themes addressed in earlier chapters. It points to key contradictions facing clinicians, to which there are few easy answers. As the NHS market develops, individual trusts, fund-holders and purchasers will want to shape their organizations and management practices to achieve the best configuration of services for patients and to secure the future of the services they are providing.

This will require different prescriptions in different places. There can be no universal remedy, no magic bullet. The management of clinical services and institutions will require the same imagination and diligence which clinicians bring to their medical work. Management will need to display the same understanding of institutional and social systems which doctors apply to the human system. This volume and those which follow it are designed to assist in the development of a deeper understanding of the structures and processes involved.

To borrow a conclusion from the strategist Robert Grant, successful management of complex organizations requires the following:

♦ objectives which are long-term, simple and agreed;
♦ a profound understanding of the competitive environment; and
♦ an objective appraisal of the available resources (Grant, 1991).

This volume is designed to help clinicians to make a step in this direction.

REFERENCES

Butler, J.R. (1992), *Patients, Policies and Politics*. Buckingham: Open University Press.
Grant, R. (1991), *Contemporary Strategy Analysis*. Oxford: Blackwell.
Health Services Journal (1994), News review, *HSJ*, 1 Sept., 6.
Klein, R. (1992), *The Politics of the National Health Service*, 2nd edn. Harlow: Longman.
Mackenzie, W.J.M. (1979), *Power and Responsibility in Health Care*. Oxford: Oxford University Press.
Watkin, B. (1978), *The National Health Service: The First Phase*. London: George Allen & Unwin.

THE IMPACT OF GOVERNMENT

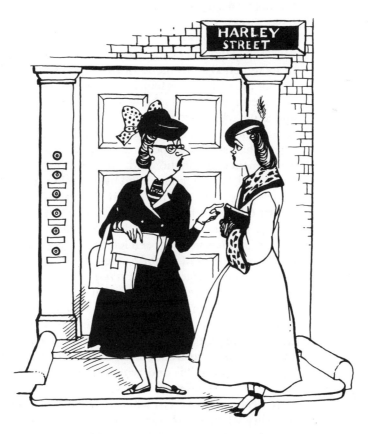

"... as I was saying to my delightful new psychiatrist ... Ever since the Health Service came in, people have been queuing up at doctors' surgeries for the sheer pleasure of it."

(First published in the *Daily Express*, 27 March 1950)

**In every developed country, health care is regarded as too
important to be left to market forces alone.**

Health care is also an expensive commodity, whether it is
accounted as a proportion of government spending or as a
percentage of the national income. It follows that it is essential to
understand the role of the government in regulating or intervening
in the arrangements for health care provision.

It is not the case that health care automatically rises to the top of
the political agenda, although as developments in the United States
have shown there may good electoral advantage in placing the
issue as a top priority. National health services are a politically
sensitive issue, and health service reforms in the UK took the form
of incremental adjustment for many years preceding the introduction of the market mechanisms for purchasing and providing.

Governments across the world have been keen to control public
spending while attempting to deny any detriment to the operational efficiency of the services whose funds are curtailed. A variety
of mechanisms have been developed with which to assess the
performance of public, and more recently, health services and
these have been accompanied by a number of *external regulators*
– including in the UK the **Audit Commission** and the **National
Audit Office**. It has been more difficult to deal with the benefits
side of the equation since the assessment of outcomes is in its
infancy and has usually been left to the judgement of professionals
or to the vagaries of performance indicators.

It has been suggested that *what gets measured gets managed,*
and it is undoubtedly the case that health authorities, threatened
with the ubiquitous league tables, have paid considerable attention
to the wishes of their political masters. It is not however the case
that government action has been entirely sector-specific and that
there are not clear trends and policies which can be traced across
ministerial portfolios and which have informed cabinet thinking
and NHS policy. In many cases procedures introduced to the NHS
have been employed elsewhere in the public sector and are part of
Treasury schemes to control expenditure or increase efficiency. *For
clinicians whose jobs entail a management responsibility, understanding the aetiology of management processes is critical to
being able to influence service development in a constructive
manner.*

If management is about successful organizational adaptation to
the environment in which an organization functions, it is important
to be able to understand the key features of that environment. The
chapter in this section focuses on the characteristics of the
environment. It looks at the ways in which health care organizations develop strategies to cope with their environment.

Andrew Gray and Bill Jenkins describe the context in which
the NHS reforms have been introduced. They show how NHS
management, both clinicians and non-clinical managers, have a

new role in the implementation of government policy. The chapter traces a distinct series of shifts in the balance of power between ministers of state, civil servants, NHS managers and the clinicians who provide medical services. The shift is exemplified in the way in which performance is defined and measured in the new NHS. *Clinicians, managers and politicians are thus embroiled in contesting a new pattern of relationships which are far from settled.* It is in this context that services are planned and developed and in which service strategies have to be worked out. Clinicians who are experienced in managerial roles will recognize many of these developments and will find a clear overview which spells out many of the interconnections and trends that are becoming apparent.

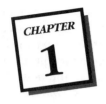

CHAPTER 1

PUBLIC MANAGEMENT AND THE NATIONAL HEALTH SERVICE

**Andrew Gray
and Bill Jenkins**

OBJECTIVES

♦ To show how developments in health care management fit within broader changes in public sector management in recent years.

♦ To understand the intentions which underpinned changes in public management and the impacts of new policies.

♦ To see how these changes influence the role of the professional staff who provide health care.

INTRODUCTION

A group of researchers enquired recently of the Department of Health whether it would be prepared to finance an evaluation of the GP **fundholder** initiative. The reply was polite and succinct, thanking the group for its interest but explaining that an evaluation was not appropriate as the initiative was now established policy. Elements of the story may be apocryphal but it does highlight a number of the characteristics and assumptions about recent development of health care in the United Kingdom: the prominence of dogma, the innovations in financial and service delivery arrangements and, for clinicians, the change in their role.

Not surprisingly, the creation of the **internal market** for health care has caused management issues to be an increasing concern of many health care professionals such as clinicians, nurses, therapists and general practitioners. For many there has been a need to learn the new vocabulary of markets and resource management dominated by such terms as competition, purchaser, contract, price, budget, added value, charters, performance indicators and quality.

These have hardly been items prominent in the curricula of medical and nursing schools. Indeed health professionals may wonder how and why the world has changed so dramatically. They would not be alone. In local government, police officers face proposals for performance related pay and short-term contracts (Cm 2280, 1993) on top of new budgeting regimes and performance indicators, head teachers find themselves 'managing' schools, and social workers compete with the private sector. In central government two-thirds of the home civil service is now employed in executive agencies, such as the infamous Child Support Agency and Prison Service, and 'managed' by chief executives via framework documents under which the agency must meet preset targets within fixed budgets. And throughout many activities are subjected to processes of 'market testing' and compulsory competitive testing (**CCT**).

Speaking of these changes, William Waldegrave, the minister then responsible for the civil service, argued that they should be seen as part of a cultural revolution increasing the accountability and quality of the public services and strengthening citizens' rights. Not all would agree. Yet how have these changes emerged? What are their strengths and weaknesses? How have they affected the changing world of UK health care?

This chapter sets out to answer these questions by, firstly, taking a broad look at the development of the new public management in the UK to identify its major characteristics and the ideas that underpin it; secondly exploring the way managerialism has evolved in the NHS from the early 1970s to the introduction of the internal market; and finally, discussing some of the major issues of concern in the public management of UK health care in the 1990s. Readers may find Box 1.1 a useful aid to navigating the various changes.

FROM PUBLIC ADMINISTRATION TO PUBLIC MANAGEMENT
In 1983 the **Griffiths Report** into the management of the NHS castigated the management and decision-making processes then operating and called for changes chiefly in the form of hierarchical line management and command and control structures (Griffiths 1983). As a result many 'administrators' at district and regional level changed their titles to 'managers', and ordered new door plates and headed notepaper. The substance of Griffiths, however, was much more than these symbolic genuflections to current fashion. Rather, it was part of a deliberate strategy to change the culture of the NHS and thus reflected a much wider movement in both the UK and elsewhere (for example Australia, New Zealand and the United States) to change both the way governments are organized and services are delivered. Indeed, two gurus of the American scene recently described the task that faces politicians and public servants in the last decade of this century as no less than 'reinventing government' (Osborne and Gaebler 1993).

Yet, in the UK, what do these reforms seek to change? Historically, the organization and delivery of government services in the UK has been characterized by two main features:

Box 1.1
A chronology of change

	Public sector developments	Health service developments
1968	Fulton committee report on Civil Service Civil Service Department set up	
1970	Central Policy Review Staff set up Programme Analysis and Review set up	
1972		Health Service reorganization (Regional, Area and District Authorities)
1975–7	Crisis of public expenditure	
1976		NHS Planning System and Resource Allocation Working Party (RAWP) established
1979	Conservative government (Mrs Thatcher) Programme Analysis and Review abandoned Efficiency Unit established	*Patients First* White Paper
1980		New management information systems (Körner) introduced
1981	Civil Service Department wound up Compulsory Competitive Tendering introduced into local government Government demands for annual efficiency savings	
1982	Financial Management Initiative	Abolition of Area Health Authorities Drive to improve internal audit
1983		Griffiths report on general management Introduction of CCT in areas such as catering and laundry services Central controls on manpower Development of performance indicators
1988	Executive Agencies announced	
1989		*Caring for People* White Paper Policy Board and NHS Management Executive established *Working for Patients* White Paper introduces internal market of purchasers and providers
1990		Community Care Act
1991	Citizen's Charter	*Health of the Nation*
1992		Patient's Charter Tomlinson Report on London's health service
1993	Sheehy report on police	

Figure 1.1
Public management as
public administration

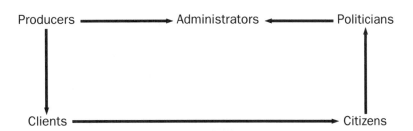

♦ the development of a career based system of public service; and
♦ the organization and delivery of services by established professionals.

In the case of central administration the ideal is a neutral, career based civil service that does the bidding of the government of the day. Based on the reforms of the Victorian Northcote Trevelyan report, this system has been one of the bastions on which the development of British government has been based (Drewry and Butcher 1991; Hennessy 1989). In a different way UK local government has also been based on a career service but, in this case, one of professional groups in associated departments (e.g. engineers, social work, housing, education).

How it was

Throughout this traditional system of public administration, politicians (ministers, members of parliament, local councillors) were separated from the delivery of service by the administrative system that 'neutrally' implemented their policies and in many instances acted as a conduit between politicians and the professional groups who delivered services to the public (see Figure 1.1; this diagram and others in this chapter are based on an idea in a paper by S. Richards, 1992). Thus, in broad terms, education was left to educators, housing to housing professionals and, of course, the delivery of medical care to health professionals, chiefly clinicians. In the 1960s and 1970s, however, a number of factors threatened this traditional method.

From the management of policy to the management of resources

Yes Minister was said to be the favourite television programme of the former prime minister, Mrs Thatcher. Any watcher of the series will recall that the main talents of Sir Humphrey Appleby, the fictional permanent secretary in the fictional Department of Administrative Affairs, were the well spoken phrase, the crafted minute and the manipulation of senior colleagues and ministers (Lynn and Jay 1982). He was good at everything and expert at nothing. Certainly the grasp of the details of financial matters was beyond him (other than expanding his departmental budget) while 'management' held no interest. Of course, the fictional minister, Jim Hacker, was if anything even more incapacitated in such matters.

As with most satire, the humour lay in exaggerating elements of the truth. As such it reflected long-held criticisms of UK central administration as wholly inadequate for present or future needs. This case was made by the 1968 Fulton Committee (Cmnd 3638, 1968) which argued forcefully for a more managerial emphasis in the UK civil service and an increased profile for personnel management and training. Early responses to the Committee included the creation of a Civil Service Department to oversee personnel matters (disbanded in 1981) and the establishment of a training body, the Civil Service College (now an executive agency).

Fulton was part of a wider reform movement that sought to introduce more rational processes of strategic planning, decision making and policy evaluation. This movement originated in arguments that the management of public expenditure in the UK was poor and uncoordinated. Consequently, in the late 1960s and early 1970s, both politicians and administrators became interested in various planning and budgeting schemas (e.g. planning, programming and budgeting (PPB) and output budgeting (OB)), as ways of introducing more rational criteria into the allocation of expenditures. These interests were given political momentum by the election of Mr Heath's government in 1970 and the introduction of reforms such as programme analysis and review (PAR) and a 'think tank' designed to assist the cabinet, the Central Policy Review Staff (CPRS) (Heclo and Wildavsky 1981; Blackstone and Plowden 1988). In local government there were also attempts to coordinate and integrate local authorities via systems of corporate management and the creation of policy and resource committees to develop council strategies, while in the health service planning systems became fashionable at both departmental and regional level.

Within a decade, however, most of these reforms had faded or failed. Two factors were central to their difficulties:

♦ the internal resistance to change; and
♦ the crisis of public expenditure of the mid 1970s.

If the former was a natural human reaction, especially to a perceived attack on privileged positions, the issue of public expenditure, however, was crucially undermining. By the mid 1970s the view of the mandarins in the Treasury was that the *use* and *consumption* of resources held little interest: traditional administrators eschewed management and especially *financial* management. What was required, therefore, was not some complex planning system but firm financial *control*. As a result, systems of *cash limits* on central departments were introduced.

This internal assessment of the state of public organizations was in tune with other movements of the time, not least those of the emerging New Right attacking the size of the state (too big) and the

Shift

effects of state expansion (the **crowding out** of the private sector and its entrepreneurial activities). This perspective also identified public organizations with inefficiencies and waste since, as monopolies, they were not subject to competition and had no incentives to hold down costs. The later years of the 1970s were therefore characterized by a shift in the focus of public administration from the management of policy to the management of resources. Sustaining this required a new culture of management.

The rise of public management

If cultural change is a matter of epistemology then the public sector has certainly been through a dramatic transformation in a decade marked not only by a change of language but also by a change in power relationships. *Hence it can be argued that the 1980s saw the demise of public administration and the rise of public management with a consequent shift in the relationships between politicians and professional groups.* This change is depicted in Figure 1.2 and can be summarized as:

◆ the redefinition or replacement of public administration by public management; and
◆ a change in the balance of power between politicians, administrators and professional groups with the evolution of a more **top-down system of control**.

The characteristics of this general model clearly vary between and within areas (civil service, local government, health services) but the overall logic of the changes of the 1980s was undoubtedly to effect a change in the *political control* of public services.

As with traditional administration, public management (or the rise of 'managerialism') is often offered as a set of neutral reforms for increasing the efficiency and responsiveness of public service delivery in a more complex economic and social environment. However, as various writers have argued, this perspective should be regarded with suspicion, not least since 'public management' carries with it its own sets of values and assumptions which if cultural change is to be achieved may be used to supplant those of the administrative and professional cultures it seeks to replace or control (Hood 1991; Pollitt 1990).

The idea, however, that the attack on the public sector and the rise of public management can be attributed to the critique of the

Figure 1.2
Public management as managerial efficiency

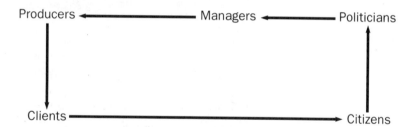

New Right and the election of Mrs Thatcher as prime minister in 1979 is, at best, partial. There were clear signs of internal moves to reform traditional administration before this time, especially in terms of installing systems of financial control into public service organizations and of raising the status and profile of 'management' as a valued activity. This said, the determination of successive Conservative governments to control public expenditure and to slim the size of the state undoubtedly provided the political impetus to drive through a reform programme. This programme was also sustained by a growing devotion to free market ideas reflected in an increasing enthusiasm for **privatization** and competition, although the development of strategies in these areas was as much the result of pragmatic policies, designed to serve varying objectives such as maximizing state revenue and massaging the size of the **public sector borrowing requirement** (PSBR), as the simple application of dogma (Marsh 1991).

In practical terms the attack on traditional public administration and the development of a management focus has a number of identifiable forms:

◆ an emphasis on economy, efficiency and effectiveness;
◆ the enhancement of delegated financial management;
◆ new personnel management systems; and
◆ a strengthening of audit through the National Audit Office and the Audit Commission.

Box 1.2
Efficiency

In central government, one strategy emerged with the establishment in 1979 of the prime minister's Efficiency Unit initially headed by Lord Rayner (Chief Executive of Marks & Spencer plc) and the evolution of a series of departmental efficiency strategies (an idea later transferred to the NHS and higher education) to identify waste and inefficiencies and correct these. Rayner's ambition was not just to make savings. His wider brief was to initiate a cultural change amongst administrators where management in general and resource management in particular would come to be seen as a valued activity if not part of the golden road to the top (Beesley 1983; Hennessy 1989; Metcalfe and Richards 1990).

The Efficiency Strategy and the Unit which it spawned (see Box 1.2) survives to this day, as does the scrutiny programme and other changes, such as management information systems for ministers (MINIS). In the mid 1980s, however, forces at the centre of government (both political and administrative) launched an altogether more ambitious programme known as the **Financial**

Management Initiative (FMI) that sought to change administrative behaviour *throughout* the departmental structure of central government. Driven by the logic as well as the intellectual baggage of management accounting, the FMI was a reform programme that set out to make 'managers at all levels' (the word *managers* was deliberately used in its publicity) accountable for the resources they used and to develop and install systems against which their performance could be measured. Accountable management therefore gave managers *budgets* for which they would be responsible and *targets* which they would agree to meet. This system was seen on the one hand to install greater control and accountability over resource use in public organizations, and on the other to have the potential to liberate managers to be entrepreneurial. That is, at least in theory, resource use was best determined by those at the grassroots level, and if 'savings' could be made then ideally they might be deployed by budget holders in ways that they thought best.

Purpose.

Yet, as various studies have demonstrated, theory may be one matter, practice is another and there is good evidence to see systems such as the FMI as being concerned first and foremost with financial controls (Gray *et al.* 1991; Humphrey *et al.* 1993). However, accountable management was intended to be part of a wider programme of change that included the development of performance indicators, management information systems and top management systems that *together* were intended to form a powerful integrated system for managing organizations from the operational level to that of strategic departmental management. *In reality only part of this materialized.*

These changes also resulted in a focus on a new system of personnel management as part of a 'results' driven organization. Traditional public administration was organized as a career service with rewards tied to the position of individuals on complex hierarchical grading structures to which were linked incremental pay spines. Promotion was generally on the basis of general job appraisals or promotion boards. The world of accountable management ushered in a different set of possibilities – in particular that of a link between reward and performance and a system where individuals were held accountable for hitting targets. It was argued that such systems, commonplace in the private sector, would transform the public sector's concern for results. It would also offer a clearer and more logical system of organizational and managerial responsibility and accountability.

Management Adv

In terms of its effect in Whitehall the FMI can be seen as a limited success (Gray *et al.* 1991). The overall influence of the philosophy that drove it, however, has been considerable. Forms of accountable management have now spread throughout the public sector in the UK and elsewhere (Humphrey *et al.* 1993). Hence in schools, hospitals, social work, the police service, the probation service and universities, budgets have been delegated, targets set and professionals designated as 'managers' with responsibilities for delivering activities and services against budgets. More importantly, these changes have made inevitable a change in the discourse of administration and professional life, with the language of financial management colonizing that of administrative and professional groups. Yet are these changes in the processes of administration enough? For those driving the reform agenda the answer to this question has been 'no'. Hence the further efforts to superimpose on the process a further set of changes that seek:

♦ to alter the structure of many public sector organizations; and
♦ to turn their orientation outwards to consumers, clients, customers and citizens.

Into the 1990s: In April 1994 London Underground experienced a spectacular two
Decentralization, hour failure during one morning rush-hour as a result of an
quality and equipment malfunction. Thousands of commuters were trapped
customer service on trains or in overcrowded stations. On resolving its difficulties London Underground apologized to its 'customers' and offered refunds to those who wished to apply for them. A day or so after this incident another set of less than enraptured customers (or clients) of another public body made their feelings known. Pressure groups of parents (mainly fathers) who found themselves targets of the Child Support Agency celebrated the first birthday of this organization by mounting demonstrations at its offices and lobbying politicians. Aside from these demonstrations, the Agency (set up to pursue absent parents and to settle 'fair' maintenance payments for dependent children) had experienced a tempestuous first year, coming under fire from various quarters including the House of Commons Select Committee on Social Services. One point made against it (but disputed by the Agency) was that as a result of the targets it had agreed to with its minister and department its activities were being directed towards easily identifiable (rather than difficult) cases. In spite of the Agency's protests many of its critics remained unconvinced.

In different ways the experiences of the London Underground and the Child Support Agency identify further strands in the development of public management that have complicated the interaction of the political, professional and managerial worlds even further (see Figure 1.3). This new set of developments is represented by:

♦ a series of *structural* reforms that have sought to distance administration and particularly service provision from political decision making;
♦ an increased emphasis on markets and competition to enhance organizational efficiency;

Figure 1.3
Public management as
customer service

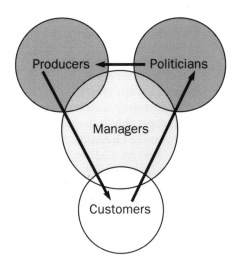

♦ a consumer-led focus that seeks to direct public services outwards to their clients as well as, in certain circumstances,
   'empowering' the clients themselves.

These themes are often entwined rather than separate, but they
also find practical expression in a series of reform initiatives that
have affected central government administration, local government
and the NHS.

In central government the main structural strategy to develop
public management has been the creation of **executive agencies**.
To this has now been added the impetus of the **Citizen's Charter**
in all its forms and, more recently, the **market testing initiative**
(Cm 1730, 1991). At the time of writing there are nearly 100
executive agencies and over two-thirds of the home civil service is
in agency form, yet the agency initiative dates back only a few years
to the Efficiency Unit Report of 1988.

The starting point for this original study was the argument
(largely unsubstantiated) that the civil service reforms detailed
above had run into the sand and that a new initiative was needed
(Davies and Willman 1991). The Efficiency Unit, under the direction of industrialist Sir Robin Ibbs, therefore conducted a study
which argued that:

♦ government was too large to be run as a single unit;
♦ the responsibility for policy and the delivery of services should
   be split; and
♦ there should be a greater focus on management, the job to be
   done and the achievement of results (Efficiency Unit 1988).

Its structural solution was the creation of departmental executive
agencies to provide discrete services within departments. Headed
by chief executives on short term contracts and performance

related reward systems, these agencies would be run at arm's length from ministers under framework documents of operational targets and budgets agreed with departments and the Treasury. Chief Executives would then be responsible for the delivery of results against targets.

After a slow start with the creation of a small number of agencies (e.g. the Vehicle Inspectorate, Companies House and the Driving and Vehicle Licensing Agency), the pace quickened as the initiative drew into its fold such giants as Social Security Benefits and such varied activities as the Historic Royal Palaces, the Stationery Office, the Meteorological Office and the Wilton Park Conference Centre (the last with only 25 staff). So far the programme illustrates a number of key aspects of the new public management:

♦ a new political environment where policy and management are seen as distinct and separate activities;
♦ a new internal managerial environment where managers are given 'freedoms' within preset frameworks and held accountable against agreed targets;
♦ a new organizational culture designed to facilitate organizational members' identification with the job, a concern with quality and a customer orientation; and
♦ a new set of personnel processes designed to enhance the above.

This is a model, therefore, of *decentralized* management within an overall system of central control. For its supporters it offers scope for the liberation of organizational energy, encouraging local initiative and entrepreneurship and enhancing greater customer or client awareness. *Yet how real freedoms can be in a system of tight expenditure controls and how entrepreneurial the behaviour within traditional public sector conceptions of accountability remain real and important questions.*

Part of the case for decentralizing public organizations is the idea that, in the past, service to clients has often been of marginal significance. This has always been a complaint of free market critics of public sector operations (e.g. **think tanks** such as the Adam Smith Institute and the Institute of Economic Affairs (IEA)) which argue that public services are monopolies with no incentives to care for their customers. This has given rise to a concern with empowering clients of public organizations and drawing them more closely into the policy process (see Figure 1.3). This has been central to initiatives in some UK local authorities, such as Tower Hamlets and York where both financial and political power have at times been decentralized, and to the Citizen's Charter (Cm 1599, 1991; see Box 1.3).

Of course, some might ask who is the **customer** of an agency such as the Child Support Agency discussed above? Is it the government (seeking to recoup public expenditure), the depen-

Box 1.3
The Citizen's Charter

> At the heart of the debate surrounding the Citizen's Charter is the question of whether the reality of its operation matches with its rhetoric in terms of issues such as:
>
> ♦ Are customers really empowered?
>
> ♦ Is the setting of service targets and performance levels a neglect of effectiveness?
>
> ♦ Who is the customer of a public organization?
>
> (Connolly *et al.* 1994; Doern 1993; Pollitt 1994)

dent child or the parents of the same? This seemingly semantic point has wider connotations not least in terms of the *political* nature of such an organization and the complexity of accountability in its operation.

charter

In the world of charters (patients, parents, travellers or electricity consumers) public management may therefore have now evolved a model of customer service dominated by a complex overlap and set of interactions between the political, professional, managerial and customer environments and spheres of responsibility (see Figure 1.3). This, in turn, may have led to new sources of legitimation in service delivery and new sets of relationships between politicians, providers and authorizers. If correct, this position is considerably removed not only from that of traditional public administration (Figure 1.1) but also from the simple and often simplistic world offered by market theorists. In this a number of characteristics are clear:

♦ The 'public' in public organization is often forgotten in a rush to follow 'good practice' (Stewart and Walsh 1992).
♦ The professional nature of many public services is often seen in a wholly negative light or as something that needs to be controlled or managed.
♦ Any form of decentralization or empowerment changes the nature of power and politics in the system.

But what of the impact of these developments and characteristics on the NHS? The remainder of this chapter will attempt to explore these.

PUBLIC MANAGEMENT AND THE NHS

Providing an efficient and effective system of health care is as much a problem for many governments at the end of the millennium as it was fifty years ago. The popularity with the general public of providing effective health care systems is undisputed. Opinion polls continue to demonstrate that health care has a high priority with voters and politicians recognize this with the claim that health care is 'safe in their hands'. Yet health care is expensive while the demand for it appears insatiable. Further, in spite of the development of universal publicly funded health care systems, inequalities persist in terms of access to treatment, development of specialties and take up of services. Hence the dream of the founders of the NHS of 'mopping up' a pool of disease and sickness has never been fulfilled. This problem became evident within a decade of the founding of the service. Since then various efforts have been made to structure and organize health care in the UK to correct perceived weaknesses and to provide a more efficient and effective service. In many ways these parallel and imitate the trends in central government outlined above, ranging from an enthusiasm for rational decision making and planning (the 1960s and 1970s), through a rush to 'managerialism' (the 1980s), to the era of the 'managed market' (the 1990s). The discussion that follows traces the logic of these developments and examines their strengths and weaknesses.

Evolution Pattern

The NHS in the 1960s and 1970s: The search for strategy and structure

Any discussion of the management of health care in the UK following the Second World War needs to recognize that while health has similarities with other areas of public policy (e.g. education, welfare) it also has significant differences. Since the creation of the NHS, health care in the UK has been primarily state funded. Although private health care practice exists (and in many ways has flourished) it is a minority actor in a larger drama where the majority of UK citizens look to the public sector for health provision and fund it out of their taxation. Health is an issue with a high profile and governments play a key role in terms of setting a framework and managing health care on a **macro level**. However, the political control of the health service on a more **micro level** is another matter since health care has been, and to a great extent is, dominated by professional groups, many of which have preserved a significant degree of autonomy. As Pettigrew *et al.* (1992) observe, hospitals and clinicians have often been seen as ideal types of a professional organization while the history of health care systems has been dominated by loose occupational coalitions struggling over the allocations of resources.

Two points are of crucial importance here:

Autonomy

◆ There is a clear pecking order amongst health care professionals with clinicians at the top of the hierarchy.

◆ The medical profession has continually acted to preserve the professionalized monopoly with regard to choices over care and treatment, justified by the sanctity of the doctor–patient relationship.

In these ways it has sought to remain professionally rather than politically or managerially accountable.

This traditional structure of the UK health care system is illustrated by Figure 1.4. *Here politicians are separated from*

Figure 1.4
Health care
management as public
administration

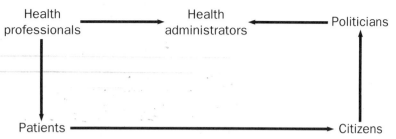

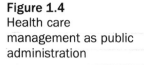

health care professionals by administrators who mediate the interaction between the two major parties. In this system the role of the political sphere is to respond to public demands, to set the framework for the organization and delivery of health care and to raise the revenue to facilitate this. These arrangements preserve professional autonomy and allow health professionals to relate to the public as patients. In such a system the role of the administrator can be seen as that of facilitator or, as Harrison has described it, as 'diplomat' (1988, Ch. 3). It was this system that dominated the early decades of the NHS and which, for a variety of reasons, came continually under pressure.

As many texts on the development of the NHS clearly point out, the structure that evolved after its creation was essentially a decentralized model loosely coordinated by the government through the Ministry of Health (Ham 1992; Levitt and Wall 1992). This system consisted of a **tripartite structure** of hospital services administered by local hospital management committees and regional hospital boards, community services administered by local health authorities and the family practitioner services. This system that was in place between 1948 and 1974 soon came under pressure most notably in terms of its failure to control the escalating costs of health care and a lack of coordination between the parts of the service. Attempts to correct these perceived malfunctions dominated the late 1960s and early 1970s.

As was noted above, two central themes of public sector reform in the 1960s and 70s were restructuring and rational planning. It should be emphasized that these are not separate activities. The advocates of rational planning and decision making often saw restructuring as a prerequisite for planning in terms of overcoming the vested interests of professional groups and the inefficiencies of fragmented organizational structures (e.g. attempts to reform local government structure and management). In the NHS these themes were manifested in:

♦ a search for a more effective and coordinated structure;
♦ efforts to rationalize the planning and resource allocation systems; and
♦ attempts to redefine and strengthen the role of management and administration.

1974 was a watershed for restructuring. It saw the culmination of a series of consultative documents and studies under first a Labour (Richard Crossman) and then a Conservative (Sir Keith Joseph) administration to produce a 'reorganized NHS' under a giant Department of Health and Social Security (Ham 1992; Harrison 1988; Holliday 1992; Levitt and Wall 1992). Under this came 14 Regional Health Authorities (RHAs) and 90 new Area Health Authorities with the majority of the latter further subdivided into Districts under District Management Teams. The intention was that this system would be more closely integrated within a strategic delivery of health care.

This intention was reinforced by the evolution of a more formalized planning (announced in *The NHS Planning System*, DHSS 1976) and efforts to place the allocation of resources between areas on a more rational and equitable basis through the development of what was known as the **RAWP formula** (named after its creator and mentor the Resource Allocation Working Party). The former was a top-down indicative planning system in which broad guidelines were set by the DHSS and passed on to the RHAs for amplification, thence to Areas and Districts which both implemented the system and fed back operational details to refine and develop the process (Harrison 1988, Ch. 2). RAWP had a different set of objectives, in particular to identify and rectify geographical disparities in funding by effecting a transfer of resources from those regions seen as 'over-provided' to those that were 'under-provided' and to develop a more strategic awareness with regard to resource use and services delivery.

This overall approach was sharpened by the attempt by the DHSS to highlight the necessity of priorities and health choices in an official document *Priorities in the Health and Personal Social Services* (DHSS 1978). This document spoke of the need to make rational choices under systems of tightening constraints and advocated planning as a 'cooperative' enterprise. It also emphasized that hard choices were necessary. However, it provided no indication of how such a system was to be implemented (Levitt and Wall 1992, Ch. 8).

As noted earlier, the nemesis of rational planning and strategic management in UK central and local government in the 1970s began with the growing economic crisis and the perceived need for different and effective systems of public expenditure constraints. This was coupled with a belief that public sector organizations paid too little attention to 'management' and were little concerned with resource use and consumption. Such fears were also mirrored in developments and the perceived 'failure' of reforms in the NHS. In particular, as Harrison and others (1988, 1992) have argued, the 'management' of the service in this period developed the following characteristics:

Bad
Management

♦ Managers were not influential actors.
♦ Health agendas were dominated by the need to react to problems rather than anticipate them.
♦ Patterns of activities and resource allocation were determined primarily by clinical judgements.
♦ Managers were producer rather than consumer orientated (i.e. patients were often marginalized).

Thus in terms of the relationships set out in the traditional system (Figure 1.4), political control over the organization and management of health care remained distant in spite of a decade of reforms. As with central government, the answer for the new generation of reformers was the amendment if not the destruction of such a cosy set of arrangements and the changing of a culture.

The NHS in the 1980s: Towards general management in health care

Bargains struck in Past

As with changes in the UK civil service and local government, it is tempting to see changes in the organization and management of health care in the 1980s as the product of a series of Conservative governments that slowly but surely applied New Right or free-market ideas to the NHS. This vision is valid only in part. To understand the developments of the 1980s (and indeed the 1990s) it is crucial to realize first that many developments represent a historical *continuity* rather than a *discontinuity* with past trends; and second that, while concerned with the implications of health care costs on public expenditure, the traditional political stance of Conservative (and often Labour) governments was to adopt a hands-off approach to the control of the health professions. The latter reflected parochial political concerns (e.g. the sympathies of professional bodies such as the British Medical Association have traditionally been to the right), and the Faustian bargain struck by Bevan in which clinicians and general practitioners were drawn into the NHS on the basis of a system of light political control and high professional autonomy.

Thus, in terms of continuities Harrison et al. argue that in the 1970s and early 1980s the political management of health care was characterized by the following:

♦ a continuity of central government financial control over overall levels of health care funding;
♦ an organizational structure based on variants of an agency type system where the centre lacked any line management control;
♦ a close (even corporatist) relationship between governments and the medical profession;
♦ a system that allowed professional groups (or at least clinical professions) to manage themselves; and
♦ a belief that better management was to be achieved through structural solutions (1992, pp. 21–6).

Whether these factors provided a satisfactory system from a political, administrative or even patient perspective is another matter. Hence the incoming Conservative government of 1979 inherited a Royal Commission Report on the NHS (the **Merrison Commission**) that while supportive of the service also argued that:

Criticisms of structure

- aspects of management were weak;
- the organizational structure contained too many tiers; and
- there was a failure to make swift and effective decisions with a consequent waste of resources (Harrison 1988, Ch. 2; Levitt and Wall 1992, Ch. 1).

The Conservative government's initial response to this was to accept the diagnosis of organizational and managerial failings and to offer its own structural solutions. These emerged in the consultative document, *Patients First* (DHSS 1979), and the subsequent reorganization of April 1982. These sought to improve the effectiveness of health care delivery by removing the area tier (created in 1974) and revamping the District Health Authorities, introducing unit management based on hospitals and streamlining the planning system. Hence, as Holliday notes, *its focus was on the devolution of control to the lowest possible levels with the argument that this would be accompanied by improvements in managerial accountability* (1992, p. 13). However, the old con-

Admin

sensus style of decision making was retained, preserving the influence of medical professionals and seeking to develop the role of administrator as 'coordinator'. At this stage, therefore, there was no clear attempt by government to develop managerial control over doctors but rather of re-engineering of the organizational system within the existing set of power relationships (Harrison 1988). This situation was soon to undergo a sea-change, however,

Management

with the publication of the Griffiths Report (1983) and the new emphasis on developing a culture of general management throughout the health service and health professions.

The origins, organizations and findings of the Griffiths Report are fully discussed elsewhere (Harrison *et al.* 1992; Holliday 1992; Levitt and Wall 1992). Nevertheless, it is worth noting here that, parallel with efforts to seek efficiency and improve management to central government, the civil service and local government, the NHS was subjected to a series of reforms that included:

- the introduction of Rayner **Efficiency Scrutinies** (1979);
- attempts to develop sophisticated and relevant management information systems (Körner Reports for DHSS from 1980);
- government demands for annual efficiency savings on budgets (1981);
- a drive to improve internal audit (1982);

- ◆ the introduction of compulsory competitive tendering (CCT) in areas such as catering and laundry services (1983);
- ◆ central controls on manpower (1983); and
- ◆ the development of **performance indicators** (1983).

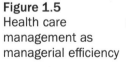

There is little evidence, however, that these formed an integrated strategy but they did reflect governmental priorities with controlling public expenditure and manpower, clamping down on waste and improving accountability. Together these shaped a climate in which Griffiths' proposals (see Box 1.4) marked a distinctive shift in the way UK health services were managed from the Department of Health to the grass roots.

In theory, if not in practice, Griffiths sought to break down the established system of organizational control in the UK health care system and replace the traditional professionally dominated consensus arrangements with a general line management in which relationships would be redefined, the status of management enhanced and, perhaps most importantly, the epistemology of management discussion amended to accord with changes elsewhere in the wider public sector discussed above (and see Figure 1.5). Thus under the Griffiths proposals the old conduit role of administrator is redefined, if not removed, to be replaced by the health manager and health management system. These are typified by top-down command and control management structures and, in the case of the DHSS itself, by an attempt to separate policy (the strategic function) from general management (administration).

The Griffiths recommendations were accepted almost in toto by the government and, at least within the DHSS, implemented with some speed as amendments were made to the Health Service Supervisory Board and the NHS Management Board. However, the first chairman of the latter, a businessman Victor Paige, resigned after two years complaining of political interference in management issues. His successor, another industrialist Len Peach (from IBM), was not asked to serve a second term and was replaced by a career NHS administrator, Duncan Nichol.

The various tensions and difficulties with these arrangements led to further revisions in 1989. The Supervisory Board was replaced by a Policy Board and the Management Board by the

Figure 1.5
Health care management as managerial efficiency

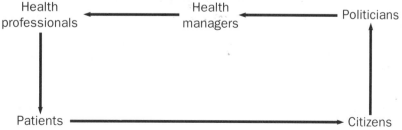

Box 1.4
The Griffiths Report

Roy Griffiths was a businessman (at that time Deputy Chairman and Managing Director of Sainsbury's plc). At the request of the Secretary of State (then Norman Fowler) he and a small team were given the brief of conducting an independent management inquiry into the NHS. This inquiry had two major foci:

♦ To examine the way in which resources were used and controlled in the NHS so as to secure the best value for money and best patient services.

♦ To identify what further management issues needed pursuing for these purposes (DHSS 1983, quoted in Harrison *et al.* 1992, p. 43).

In the style of Rayner scrutinies, the inquiry was short and sharp and produced a report only some 25 pages in length. Its analysis, however, was biting and forceful. It argued that:

♦ Individual management accountability could not be clearly identified.

♦ The machinery of implementation was weak.

♦ There was a lack of a performance orientation and little evaluation of health care activities.

♦ Little attention was paid to consumers.

The Griffiths recommendations were:

♦ A Health Service Supervisory Board should be created in the DHSS (chaired by the minister, but also including non-executive members with managerial skills and experience) to oversee NHS strategy.

♦ Directly under this should come a multi-disciplinary Management Board responsible for the implementation of this strategy (this should encompass all major NHS managerial responsibilities and in particular personnel management).

♦ Consensus management should be abolished and general line management introduced throughout the NHS (i.e. at Regional, District and Unit level).

♦ Clinicians were to be encouraged to participate in management and in particular to be held responsible for resources consumed ('resource management').

♦ A greater emphasis should be placed on patients and 'community' opinion (Harrison 1988, pp. 60–3; Harrison *et al.* 1992, pp. 41–7).

NHS Management Executive (NHSME) and Duncan Nichol's title changed to Chief Executive. *In this new regime the distinction between policy and management is enhanced.* The Policy Board (with political, civil service, NHS, medical and external members) was charged with advising the Secretary of State on the formation, implementation and evaluation of NHS policies. In particular, its task was to set objectives for the NHSME. In turn the NHSME was charged with moving the NHS in the directions set by government policy. However, to see the role of the NHSME as divorced from policy would be an error. Its major functions now include:

Changes

♦ setting objectives for the NHS (within the remit of broader policy); and
♦ monitoring results of both a long and short term nature (e.g. integration of primary and secondary care, development of effectiveness measures, waiting list management, and overall financial management).

In theory at least, the post-Griffiths system at the DHSS (and later the Department of Health) was intended to move politicians into a more strategic role and to develop an arm's length relationship between political (and strategic) and operational management issues. Whether this is realistic remains open to question. Indeed, Griffiths himself speaking in 1991 was less than happy with subsequent developments. Arguing that the top level changes had been 'correct in concept', he complained that they had been 'half hearted in implementation'. In particular, there had been 'no attempt to establish objectives at the centre and no concentration on outcomes' (quoted in Harrison *et al*. 1992, p. 62).

Rhetoric?

The introduction of general management in the lower reaches of the service followed after a short period of consultation but with mixed effects. Harrison et al. note, 'it has often been taken for granted that the Griffiths changes to NHS management represent a revolutionary development from past practice. The grounds on which this assertion is made are often unstated' (1992, p. 47). Drawing on their own and other research, these authors argue that the characteristics of post-Griffiths changes were management agendas dominated by financial matters (often to the detriment of patients) and little evidence of management (other than in exceptional circumstances) actively challenging clinicians. Similarly, the latter generally showed little interest in participating in the management process (unless their direct interests were threatened) and a similar lack of enthusiasm for taking on responsibilities for resource management. There was little evidence of cultural change but plenty 'of the old NHS tribalism', while 'a proactive management, setting goals, implementing plans for their achievement and monitoring progress remained a vision rather than a reality' (Harrison 1988, p. 65).

Old Rituals Die Hard.

The reasons for these difficulties are seen to emerge from

tensions that existed within the Griffiths model as well as failure to recognize specific characteristics of the NHS likely to constrain the reforms' impact. In particular it is argued that:

- Griffiths offered a vision of managerialism that is based on distrust in contrast to the professionally based system of consensus management it replaced.
- The model assumed that political and managerial matters are different and separable.
- There was an assumption that health care objectives can (or will) be clearly defined at departmental and political levels.

The question is, therefore, whether the Griffiths reforms were more style than substance and whether, before 1989 at least, there was any evidence of true cultural change in the NHS and erosion of professional dominance. *Undoubtedly some considered that further moves were needed to move health care into a more competitive world to strengthen the managerial changes that Griffiths had set under way. This meant markets, prices and contracts.*

Griffiths Prompted significant change

The NHS in the 1990s: Markets, managers and professionals

At the end of 1992, Channel 4 Television broadcast a documentary series on King's Healthcare in London during its first year as a NHS trust. The main themes of these programmes were 'management, medics and money'. The series depicted the hospital struggling desperately to manage its finances in the new NHS internal market. It also stressed the sharp conflicts between the new management regime of the trust headed by its Chief Executive and many of the clinicians working in the hospital. Further, it noted that the clinicians were also sometimes divided amongst themselves especially with regard to the rights of newly appointed 'clinical directors' to control the work and activities of their colleagues.

King's can be seen on the one hand as a uniquely hard pressed hospital struggling to cope at a particular point in time. On the other hand, it may also be seen as a microcosm of much that has been happening in the NHS especially during the teething difficulties of the internal market. These include:

- a new political environment of health care;
- a new managerial environment that goes beyond Griffiths;
- a new professional environment;
- a new culture (imposed and created); and
- new processes within health care organizations.

workers as Managers

This has led to new sets of relationships in health care organizations as shown in Figure 1.6. In this new world the old orders have changed in a complex and shifting fashion. In particular not only does 'management' now affect directly professional, political and patient behaviour but these groups in different but significant ways are being drawn into the 'management' process. Indeed, the term

Figure 1.6
Health care
management as
customer service

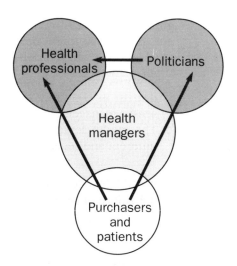

'managed market', often used to describe the current (i.e. 1994)
situation in health care, is open to different and subtle connotations; e.g. is the market being managed at the political level or has it
become dominated by management rhetoric and values to the
detriment of professional perspectives on health care? We return to
these questions below. First, however, it is necessary to identify the
major features of the current situation and examine how it came
about.

The literature on the creation and development of the NHS
internal market is thin but growing (Butler 1992, 1993; Holliday
1992). Whether it shows a revolution or paradigm shift in the
management of health care in the UK (Holliday 1992) is a matter of
debate. As a change in the delivery of a set of major public services,
however, its comprehensiveness and speed of implementation are
not in doubt. Surprisingly, the origins of these changes appear to
have been almost the product of a series of policy accidents rather
than a planned political strategy. Hence pressures on the NHS in the
late 1980s resulted in Mrs Thatcher deciding to review the service.
In mid flow this review switched its focus from the funding of
health care and different modes of its provision to an organizational
and managerial one – could the service be organized in a more
efficient way? At this point the views of New Right think tanks and
health economists gained the ascendancy, coming to fruition in the
publication in 1989 of *Working for Patients* (Cm 555).

Working for Patients introduced to the NHS a more sophisticated version of the purchaser–provider model already trialed in
changes to service delivery in local government. This model was
later developed in the Next Steps initiative in central government
(see above) and in other areas such as community care, education
and housing (Taylor-Gooby and Lawson 1993). In essence the
purchaser–provider split seeks to introduce competition into

public sector organizations and to increase efficiency by separating out the purchaser and provider roles. The NHS case, however, is much more comprehensive than earlier efforts being part of a larger plan to create a comprehensive internal market in health care.

As Harrison *et al.* (1992) have argued, the main post-Griffiths problems were perceived by the government and by other influential groups not only outside but also within the NHS itself, as including:

◆ the dominance of macro-financial issues;
◆ the failure of attempts to secure internal financial controls (e.g. clinical budgeting);
◆ the continuity of in-built problems (e.g. waiting lists, geographical disparities such as over-provision of clinical services in London); and
◆ a superficial concern with patients ('consumers').

Working for Patients sought to tackle some (but by no means all) of these by the creation of an internal market where health purchasers and providers of secondary and community health care would be split and linked by contracts. In this new world, purchasers would be District Health Authorities (DHAs), GP fundholders and private patients. Providers would be hospitals, NHS trusts and private sector organizations. The two new key players in the contracting game were GP fundholders and trusts. GP fundholders were practices which, having met certain criteria (size of lists, organization, etc.), could apply for budgets to purchase patient care and thus become autonomous actors in the market process. Trusts were organizations (usually hospitals or groups of hospitals) which opted out of control by DHAs to become independent self-governing bodies with the capacity to set their own terms and conditions for staff remuneration and sell their services to public and private health clients. They were to be governed by Boards of Directors and accountable directly to the DHSS. Their revenue would be derived directly from the sale of their services.

These changes were implemented as part of the National Health Service and Community Care Act (1990). Since then successive waves of reform in each financial year have led to the majority of large hospitals being awarded trust status and a significant number of GPs as fundholders. As might have been anticipated, however, these changes have not been without controversy. Criticisms have focused on:

◆ escalating numbers of managers and management costs (the Secretary of State for Wales called for 'more operations, not slogans; and medicines, not glossy leaflets';

[handwritten margin notes: Problems of the Past. / Purchasers Providers who's who? / Criticisms New Managers]

- the emerging two-tier system of patient treatment resulting from the introduction of GP fundholders, the budgetary restrictions and consequent closure of hospital beds;
- the lack of accountability of trusts and their internal operating procedures including secrecy, management styles and, in a minority of cases, financial mismanagement.

Defence

But supporters of the reforms have accused the DHSS of failing to give trusts the freedoms they promised, of interfering in the operation of the internal market (e.g. the case of health care in London) and of maintaining centralized systems of setting the salaries of professional groups (e.g. clinicians and nurses) when the logic of the trust system is to decentralize pay and rewards.

In four years (1990-94) the organization of health care delivery in the UK has been changed more radically than at any time since its inception. Much of this can be attributed to *Working for Patients.* But to understand the continually changing environment of health care one must also note:

Reasons For Change

- changes in Community Care implemented in 1991;
- health targets as set out in *Health of the Nation* (Cm 1523, 1991);
- consumerism and the Patient's Charter (1992);
- the debate over health care in London (the **Tomlinson Report** 1992; *Making London Better*).

Pass The Buck

Most of these extend the purchaser–provider model to the public services, add to the growing rhetoric (if not the reality) of consumerism and reveal the distinctions (economic, geographical and professional) that make the realization of markets difficult. In the case of community care, for example, a continuing problem has been the link between the health services and the personal social services, in particular the responsibility and provision for mental illness, mental handicap and geriatric care.

The continuing difficulties to find solutions in this area led the government to turn again to Roy Griffiths. His report was the basis of *Caring for People* (DHSS 1989) and subsequent community care legislation. As with other initiatives, the government sought to install greater delegated financial management into this area and, via the development of the purchaser–provider split, more choice, flexibility and innovation in care delivery. The key terms were again value-for-money, efficiency, accountability and quality.

These changes reorganized and redirected local government social service departments. However, the development of this new regime in parallel with the internal health care market placed further strains on health care organizations. Meanwhile, other pressures have arisen from the advance of consumerism, in

Other Problems

particular the commitments of the Patient's Charter to waiting times, as well as from the government's publication in *Health of the Nation* of a key series of **health targets** (e.g. for heart disease, obesity, cancers, smoking related illnesses). As many have noted, such political commitment to public health and its promotion is commendable but it also places further pressures on the changing health care system.

It is very much a moot point whether the internal market has led to the erosion of professional dominance and the rise of managerialism. In the appointment of Alan Langlands from within the NHSME to succeed Duncan Nichol as chief executive, and the recent streamlining of the regions as the precursor for their eventual replacement by the Department's own regional offices, some have seen the triumph of a new order of managed competition in health care with the NHSME at the centre. Some professionals maintain that to secure their positions in the new world, they must themselves take on the role of manager. Others deny this. What is clear, however, is that different sorts of organizations and participants have emerged in health care.

SUMMARY

This chapter has sought to place the developments in the management of British health care into a context of change and reform of public service management in general. Undoubtedly the changes have placed an emphasis on efficiency, competition and consumer choice. This has brought new sources of legitimation and rationing in service delivery, new relationships between providers and authorizers or purchasers, new codes of accountability and a more fragmented delivery service.

The organizations providing the care have changed almost out of all recognition in a very short time. The Department of Health itself has been transformed and the Regional Health Authorities and Special Health Authorities remain only to oversee the end of their hitherto distinctive functions. New organizational forms, notably trusts (and now mergers of trusts) and consortia of general practitioners, are active in seeking to influence the new internal market. If once the organizational pattern could be described as homogeneous and stable, that must now give way to heterogeneous and dynamic.

Similarly, the processes which characterize health care delivery have been revolutionized. The jargon is now of strategic directions, market positioning, resource management, and flexible response. There is a volcano of new regimes of decentralized responsibility and accountability, systems of cash constraints on programmes and activities, strategies for human resource management, and programmes for quality assurance. Not surprisingly, this has been accompanied by a rapid rise in the size of the management cadre. Yet the professionals have found that they are now more actively involved, like it or not (and many do not), in the management of their institutions. Marketing, for example, has become not only a key activity for the new organizations but also a central function for health care professionals, not excluding consultants.

The criteria for a health care organization have also changed. More prominent now are value-for-money (i.e. economy and efficiency) as well as effectiveness. More attention is paid to the quality of service before and after the actual treatment. Thus managers focus not only on waiting lists but also on waiting times. Moreover, new proposals for changes in regimes of clinical care must be supported by cost advantages if they are to be successful in even appearing on policy agendas.

Yet, we may ask how much of this is substance and how much mere form. There are signs that the much vaunted internal market has given way to a system of managed competition (managed, that is, by the Department), that new business plans and strategy documents are essentially political responses to pacify the NHSME rather than expressions of principle to guide institutional actions. It is certainly easy to be cynical after discussing these changes with managers and professionals at the point of service delivery. However, there *are* undoubted signs of major substantive change. The chosen instruments, for example, have altered the nature of power and politics in the health service. This has been at the expense of the professionals and to the advantage of the managers. It is the latter whose position in the interaction between patients, purchasers, politicians and professionals is now pivotal to health care.

Whether all this is to the benefit of patient well-being and the health of the nation is hotly disputed. But it is a testament to a commitment to implementation. However, it has only just begun and, as the following chapters demonstrate, there remain major issues to resolve.

FURTHER READING

Those interested in the debate on the changing management of the NHS can refer to publications such as *The Health Service Journal* and the comment, news and educational sections of *The British Medical Journal*. General issues here include the effects of implementing the internal market via trusts and GP fundholders. More specific problems such as performance indicators in health care, hospital league tables, the management of finance versus the treatment of patients, and new systems of pay and conditions in health care organization, are also covered widely in the national press, in professional publications and in journals such as *The Economist*. Examples of compendia of these publications include those of the *British Medical Journal*. Anyone with access to wider library resources will also find these issues examined in journals such as *Public Administration, Financial Accountability and Management*, and *Public Money and Management*.

> More wide-ranging examinations of the management changes, both in general and in the NHS, are available in:
>
> ◆ British Medical Journal (1991), *The Health of the Nation*. BMJ Books, London.
>
> ◆ British Medical Journal (1992), *The Future of Health Care*. BMJ Books, London.
>
> ◆ British Medical Journal (1992), *The Health Debate Live*. BMJ Books, London.
>
> ◆ British Medical Journal (1993), *London after Tomlinson*. BMJ Special Publication, London.
>
> ◆ Flynn, N. (1992), *Public Sector Management*, 2nd edn, Harvester Wheatsheaf, Hemel Hempstead.
>
> ◆ Ham, C. (1992), *Health Policy in Britain*, 3rd edn, Macmillan, London.
>
> ◆ Pollit, C. (1992), *Managerialism and the Public Services*, Blackwell, Oxford.

REFERENCES

Beesley I. (1983), The Rayner Scrutinies. In: Gray, A.G. and Jenkins, W.I. (Eds), *Policy Analysis and Evaluation in British Government*. London: RIPA.

Blackstone, T. and Plowden, W. (1988), *Inside the Think Tank: Advising the Cabinet 1971–83*. London: William Heinemann.

Butler, J.R. (1992), *Patients, Policies and Politics*. Buckingham: Open University Press.

Butler, J.R. (1993), A case study of the National Health Service: Working for patients. In: Taylor-Gooby, P. and Lawson, R. (Eds) *Markets and Managers: New Issues in the Delivery of Welfare*, Buckingham: Open University Press.

Cm 555 (1989), *Working for Patients*. London: HMSO.

Cm 1523 (1991), *The Health of the Nation*. London: HMSO.

Cm 1599 (1991), *The Citizen's Charter: Raising the Standard*. London: HMSO.

Cm 1730 (1991), *Competing for Quality*. London: HMSO.

Cm 2280 (1993), *Inquiry into Police Responsibilities and Rewards* (The Sheehy Report). London: HMSO.

Cmnd 3638 (1968), *Report on the Committee on the Civil Service* (Ch. Lord Fulton). London: HMSO.

Connolly, M., McKeown, P. and Milligan-Byrne, G. (1994), Making the public sector user friendly? A critical examination of the citizens charter, *Parliamentary Affairs*, 47:1.

Davies, A. and Willman, J. (1991), *What Next? Agencies, Departments and the Civil Service*. London: Institute for Public Policy Research.

DHSS (1976), *The NHS Planning System*. London: DHSS.

DHSS (1978), *Priorities in the Health and Personal Social Services*. London: DHSS.

DHSS (1979), *Patients First*. London: DHSS.

DHSS (1989), *Caring for People*. London: DHSS.

Doern, G.B. (1993), The UK citizen's charter: origins and implementation in three agencies, *Policy and Politics*, 21:1.

Drewry, G. and Butcher, T. (1991), *The Civil Service Today*, 2nd edn. Oxford: Blackwell.

Efficiency Unit (1988), *Improving Management in Government: The Next Steps*. London: HMSO.

Flynn, N. (1992), *Public Sector Management,* 2nd edn. Hemel Hempstead: Harvester Wheatsheaf.

Gray, A.G. and Jenkins, W.I., with Flynn, A.C. and Rutherford, B.A. (1991), The management of change in Whitehall: the experience of the FMI, *Public Administration*, 69:1.

Griffiths, R. (1983), *NHS Management Inquiry*. London: Department of Health and Social Security.

Ham, C. (1992), *Health Policy in Britain*, 3rd edn. London: Macmillan.

Harrison, S. (1988), *Managing the National Health Service: Shifting the Frontier*. London: Chapman & Hall.

Harrison, S., Hunter, D., Marnoch, G. and Pollitt, C. (1992), *Just Managing: Power and Culture in the National Health Service*. London: Macmillan.

Heclo, H. and Wildavsky, A. (1981), *The Private Government of Public Money*, 2nd edn. London: Macmillan.

Hennessy, P. (1989), *Whitehall*. London: Seeker & Warburg.

Holliday, I. (1992), *The NHS Transformed*. Manchester: Baseline Books.

Hood, C. (1991), A public management for all seasons? *Public Administration*, 69:1.

Humphrey, C., Miller, P. and Scapens, R.W. (1993), Accountability and accountable management in the UK public sector, *Accounting, Auditing and Accountability*, 6:3.

Levitt, R. and Wall, A. (1992), *The Reorganized National Health Service*, 4th edn. London: Chapman & Hall.

Lynn, J. and Jay, A. (1982), *Yes, Minister*. London: BBC Books.

Marsh, D. (1991), Privatization under Mrs Thatcher: a review of the literature, *Public Administration*, 69:4.

Metcalfe, L. and Richards, S. (1990), *Improving Public Management*, 2nd edn. London: Sage Publications.

Osborne, D. and Gaebler, T. (1993), *Reinventing Government*. New York: Plume Books.

Pettigrew, A., Ferlie, E. and McKee, L. (1992), *Shaping Strategic Change: Making Change in Large Organizations—the Case of the National Health Service*. London: Sage Publications.

Pollitt, C. (1990), *Managerialism and the Public Services*. Oxford: Blackwell.

Pollitt, C. (1994), The Citizen's Charter: a preliminary analysis, *Public Money and Management*, 14(2):9–14.

Richards, S. (1992), *Who Defines the Public Good? The Consumer Paradigm in Public Management*. London: Public Management Foundation.

Stewart, J. and Walsh, K. (1992), Change in the management of public services, *Public Administration,* 70:4.

Taylor-Gooby, P. and Lawson, R. (Eds) (1993), *Markets and Managers: New Issues in the Delivery of Welfare.* Buckingham: Open University Press.

ACKNOWLEDGE-MENT The authors gratefully acknowledge S. Richards as the source of a key theme used throughout this chapter.

SECTION II

KEY PERSPECTIVES IN NHS MANAGEMENT

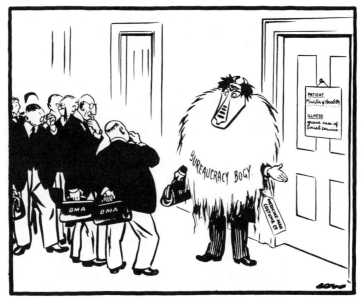

"... But do you think it will cure the patient?"

(First published in the *Evening Standard*, 19 May 1944)

While government plays a significant role in setting many of the parameters within which health care services are delivered, there remains an important task for local management owing to the particularity of local needs, the variability of available resources and capabilities, and the rapid pace of technological and other developments.

Any choice of 'lenses' with which to view this field is bound to be idiosyncratic. The editors have tried to identify approaches which are distinct and important in the pattern of decisions and actions which determine the shape of health care services. The chapters in this section cover major sets of initiatives which have been undertaken at most, if not all, levels of the service. In each there have been government initiatives aimed at increasing efficiency, or accountability, or simply improving the quality of the services provided. Clinical managers can be expected to be concerned with each of these areas and will benefit from a sound review of the particular field.

Aims

The authors describe the developments in their particular field and also the key dilemmas which need to be resolved if clinicians and managers are to develop effective services within the NHS market. Starting with the development and implementation of strategy, the section covers the management of money and people, closing with a review of the contentious and complex issue of quality.

The NHS has always had policies but what do we mean by strategy? Within a centrally planned NHS the key questions of coordination and efficiency came to the fore. By the use of planning procedures and the central directives of the Department of Health, clinicians and managers could be clear of what was expected from them and how they were to fit into the comprehensive national service. Problems of disagreements could be dealt with by reference to a higher level of administrative authority and the rights of doctors and other staff were safeguarded. The market has changed this centralized process to one which focuses on the ability of the independent hospital trust or fundholder to win contracts and to innovate so as to find the most cost-effective ways of meeting their contracted obligations.

This requires the development of new capabilities, particularly among the senior staff and management boards of trusts. While they remain subject to external scrutiny, they do have significant new freedoms provided they are able to ensure that departments and services remain effective and viable. Trusts, purchasers and general practices are concerned with identifying viable plans with which to coordinate their efforts and to make the most of the funds which are available for treating patients. Often the contents of these plans are largely determined by history and local circumstances. The major criticism of planning in the NHS has been that implementation has seldom followed as the plans implied. While

Waste of time

Sonterous

20-1-02

this does not, of itself, necessarily mean that such plans were completely worthless, it does mean that in some places the planning forums were perceived as talking shops in which important issues were raised but seldom settled.

The creation of board-like structures within the NHS suggests the importation of commercial and business procedures from the private sector, but are they likely to prove any more successful given the political and economic realities with which the NHS has to live? **David Hunter** provides a guide to a contentious field, pointing to the wide variety of approaches and the limitations of existing evidence about effective strategy making.

These economic realities lead us to a major focus of attention in NHS management – namely the **management of money**. Frequently the root cause of NHS problems is put down either to the lack of finance or to its inappropriate use.

- ◆ What are the procedures and mechanisms with which finance is made available and managed within the NHS?
- ◆ How are processes to ensure audit and accountability managed and are there any tools with which alternative proposals for the use of funds can be evaluated?

One of the first management processes which any clinician has to understand is the allocation, budgeting and control of finance, and **John Glynn** provides a broad review of these processes within the context of active service management.

The majority of revenue funds in most service industries is spent on staff and the NHS is no exception. The clinical manager has to manage staff or contract with external firms and agencies who provide staff when they are required. There are many serious limitations within which managers of clinical services are forced to work which make this process more difficult. **Alison Baker and David Perkins** point to the changes that have accompanied the introduction of the market. In particular, they address the shift from central determination of manpower requirements and management processes to the broad principle that those who are responsible for the provision of services should determine their staffing needs and that they should vary the mix of staff to meet operational requirements and secure cost-effective services.

The objective of strategy, financial management and management of staff is to provide high-quality services efficiently. This section ends with a review of the question of **quality** and the processes which are used to ensure and to assess quality. While the vast majority of clinical staff have very clear views of what constitutes quality in the individual patient intervention, this does not necessarily imply that the service provided to a community is of high quality. For instance a community trust may provide a very high quality of psychotherapy to those patients who are admitted to the programme, but what of those who are excluded owing to lack of funds or a lack of awareness that the service exists. While we are used to the measurement of quality in other fields this is still an underdeveloped science in the field of health care management. **Barbara Morris and Louise Bell** provide a comprehensive review of the field, focusing on development within the NHS and pointing to new possibilities for securing and measuring quality.

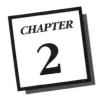

CREATING HEALTH SERVICES STRATEGY

David J. Hunter

OBJECTIVES

♦ To show how strategic management has evolved since the NHS reforms of April 1991.

♦ To examine the factors which influence the creation of strategy and those which constrain its development and implementation.

♦ To see how different strands of the NHS contribute to the strategy of the service and how their contributions influence the whole.

INTRODUCTION

The 1991 NHS reforms have resulted, in theory at least, in overturning the management style and strategic orientation which influenced the development of health policy and health strategy in the decade between 1974 and 1984. There then followed a short interregnum, from the mid-1980s until the reform proposals appeared in the 1989 White Paper, *Working for Patients*, during which traditional conceptions of strategic management and planning were addressed and reshaped in the context of what has been called 'new public management' (Hood 1991).

The purpose of this chapter is to offer a critical appraisal of the strategic function as it has evolved since the NHS reforms were implemented in April 1991. It focuses on the purchaser–provider separation and describes and assesses how in each sector the key stakeholders are creating strategy. As part of the assessment, the factors and influences promoting and constraining the creation of strategy are considered. It is, of course, not possible at this stage of the reform process to offer a definitive account of what is happening. The changes continue to unfold and the policy landscape is subject to constant shifts. However, the material presented does illustrate the complexity of what is happening and the difficulty of regarding strategy in anything other than dynamic and emergent rather than planned or deliberate terms.

The chapter is in five sections. The first section examines the term 'strategy' and offers a definition to guide the subsequent discussion and analysis. The second charts the development of strategy within the NHS over two time periods: between 1974 and 1984, and from 1989 to the present, covering the period of the post-1989 NHS and community care reforms. This brief scene-setting section is important in demonstrating the enormity of the challenge presented by the 1991 reforms and the break with accepted notions of strategy development and health planning which they represent. There then follow separate sections on strategic development in purchaser agencies and in provider units respectively. A final section seeks to draw the different strands together and assess the place of strategy in the new NHS and community care settings, and makes some interim observations about progress and likely future directions.

WHAT IS STRATEGY?

Traditionally in the British NHS and elsewhere strategy has been seen as top-down, rational and formal. This was certainly the case between 1974 and 1984 as we shall see in the next section. Such a conception of strategy had its counterpart in the command and control, top-down notion of management which was to the fore in public policy during the 1970s.

A revised, and rather more complex, conception of strategy has been propounded by Mintzberg (1990) and other writers. This develops the idea of strategy as a *process* as well as an *outcome*. Mintzberg writes of an 'emergent strategy', in contrast to a 'deliberate strategy', by which he means a series of actions converging into a pattern or series of patterns. The actions may become deliberate if the pattern is recognized and then legitimized by senior management but this is a *post hoc* rationalization of what has emerged organically. Other forms of strategy fall between the two extremes of deliberate and emergent and combine deliberation and control with flexibility and organizational learning.

There are therefore different perspectives on what strategy really is. For example, Johnson (1987) has identified three views of the strategic management process:

◆ a rationalistic view of strategic management in which strategy is seen as the outcome of a sequential, planned search for optimal solutions to defined problems;
◆ an adaptive or incremental view of strategic management which evolves in an additive pattern;
◆ an interpretive view in which strategy is seen as the product of individual or collective sense making.

Pettigrew, Ferlie and McKee (1992) draw a distinction in the public sector between policy and strategy. They argue that histori-cally there has been a greater emphasis on 'policy' (content) than 'strategy' (content and process) but that there is now increasing interest in the application of the strategy literature to health care settings. The notion of NHS general managers, when they were introduced in 1983 following implementation of the Griffiths reforms, as potential strategists was developed by Parston (1986) and is closely associated with Evans' work. Evans' (1987a,b) view was that in order to achieve a high rate of service change policy development was by itself insufficient. It was the role of senior management to develop a coherent style which could lead to strategies for change across the organization.

As Baeza *et al.* (1993) observe, although a useful concept, strategy remains problematic because of a lack of consensus over its precise meaning. Notwithstanding this lack of consensus over the meaning of strategy, it is possible to find general agreement on the fact that the classical literature on strategy dating from the 1960s and 1970s was based on the idea of the heroic leader or manager who lead decisively from the top of the organization, inspired his (or less commonly, her) colleagues, and achieved successful implementation with little deviation along the way. Such a conception was more a product of Taylor's 'scientific management' body of theory and machine-like notions of how organizations work rather than a reflection of the reality of organizational life at this, or any other, time.

In challenging this rather mechanistic and simplistic view of strategy, Mintzberg's notion of strategy as the result of a myriad of decisions and not the logical or inevitable outcome of economic and technical rationality is akin to the bureaucratic politics view of organizational life most ably articulated by Allison (1971). Mintzberg (1988, p. 14) defines strategy as what organizations actually achieve and not just that which they intend to achieve. 'Defining strategy as a plan in advance of taking action is not sufficient.'

In understanding the creation of strategy in any organization, including the NHS, it is therefore necessary to move away from the corporate planning models prevalent in the 1960s and 1970s, with their emphasis on synoptic rationality, and to look at what managers actually do in the strategic direction of their particular enterprise rather than at what might be done in any prescriptive sense.

For the purposes of this chapter, then, strategy is perceived as being 'contingent on both the *nature of the organization* (its size, its value system, its degree of specialization) and *its external environment* (stable, unstable)' (McKevitt 1992, p. 35). In this conception, strategy could be seen as a continuum with deliberate, planned strategy at one end and emergent strategy at the other. Given the uncertainty that has swept through the public sector, and is still sweeping through much of it, over the past decade or so, the idea of a clear means–ends relationship in policy making, if indeed it ever did resemble practice, is seen to belong to what might be termed the 'Jurassic Park' school of management thinking. It is arguable that strategy development in the NHS has never achieved the ideal of corporate rationality beloved of the architects of the 1974 NHS reorganization. Indeed, arguably it was the failure of this rational, comprehensive model of planning that led to widespread disillusionment with planning and eventually to the various reform moves in the 1980s culminating in the 1989 White Paper (Barnard 1991). It was certainly a factor in the various developments that took place over this period as policy makers sought a way of trying to square the circle of rising demand for health care coupled with finite resources. Barnard (1991, p. 136) sees the failure of this particular form of central planning as 'perhaps the most significant feature of the intellectual debate in public policy' and as having paved the way for 'the school of thought which in many countries enjoyed ascendency during the past decade (with its) reaffirmation of the superiority of markets and price mechanisms as the means of satisfying human wants'.

Mkt Supreme mentality.

The 1991 NHS reforms overturned the corporate rationalist approach, replacing it with the notion of business rationality, or managed competition, although as McKevitt (*ibid.*) argues, the reforms were not so much concerned with high level strategy as with business level or operational changes (see Figure 2.1). Health care reform in the UK has not been about finding policy solutions

Figure 2.1
Levels of strategy

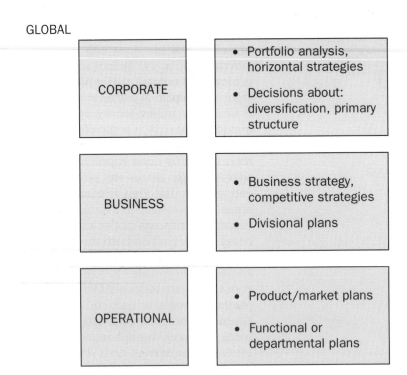

GLOBAL

CORPORATE
- Portfolio analysis, horizontal strategies
- Decisions about: diversification, primary structure

BUSINESS
- Business strategy, competitive strategies
- Divisional plans

OPERATIONAL
- Product/market plans
- Functional or departmental plans

LOCAL

Source: McKevitt
(1992, p. 44)

Real Goal?

to basic strategic questions such as who is to benefit, at what cost, and with what safeguards for the disadvantaged in society. It has been chiefly about technical and operational issues concerning the most efficient way of delivering health care.

To locate the strategic issues means going back to the **1946 Health Act** which sets out the objectives of the NHS. These were revisited by the 1979 Royal Commission on the NHS but since then have not figured prominently in government policy statements on health issues. This is not to suggest that there is an absence of strategy. Indeed, since 1991 there has been a rash of strategies including the health strategy (Cm 1986, 1992), the research and development strategy (DoH 1991, 1993b), and initiatives linked to the Patient's Charter. But, possibly with the exception of the health strategy, these are less about grand or corporate strategy and more about business and operational strategies such as achieving improved efficiency and effectiveness in terms of what currently is done by way of health service delivery and health promotion. Indeed, there are doubts about the extent to which there is an overall corporate strategy for the NHS linking the separate strategies, or whether it is a case of discrete strategies having been spawned for separate reasons which may or may not cohere.

In the next section we turn to a deeper analysis of the differing conceptions of strategy in the NHS in the period 1974 to 1984, and then from 1989 to the present.

THE EVOLUTION OF HEALTH STRATEGY

In this section, two periods of health strategy development are described. In order better to understand the creation of health strategy following the 1991 NHS reforms, it is helpful to provide a brief comment on developments in the period before the reforms in which the pursuit of strategy took a rather different form – and one which has not entirely disappeared.

Whether the different approaches to strategy development represented by these respective stages in the development of the NHS are superior to one another in any way is arguable. At the end of the day, the NHS remains as it always has been, an organization which is accountable to the Secretary of State for Health and, through her or him, to Parliament. There is, therefore, a high degree of centralization and control from the top despite the rhetoric over many years in favour of devolved management and local responsibility. Accountability remains firmly upwards both in respect of purchasers and providers. The Functions and Manpower Review, the conclusions of which were announced in late 1993, largely confirm this view (Hunter 1993a). National strategy, therefore, is ultimately articulated by Ministers, advised by the NHS Policy Board, by the Department of Health policy divisions, and the NHS Executive which is itself part of the Department.

**Health Strategy,
1974–1984**

*Initial
Planning*

The 1974 NHS reorganization represented the first major attempt to improve strategic management in the Service. Since then the NHS has undergone three further major reorganizations. The 1974 reorganization was principally informed by notions of inducing greater rationality into processes of health planning and priority setting in what was then a unified service in respect of purchaser and provider functions. The 1962 Hospital Plan was the first early example of national planning but it was not until 1976, when the Department issued a consultative document on priorities for health and personal social services, that an attempt was made 'to establish rational and systematic priorities throughout the health and personal social services' (DHSS 1976, p. 1). The document was principally aimed at securing commitment to community care, which was generally considered to be preferable to long-stay institutional care, whether in hospital or residential homes, for the so-called priority groups – namely, mentally ill, mentally and physically handicapped, and elderly people. Current policy is informed by virtually the same beliefs and commitment to community care alternatives to institutional care (Cm 849, 1989).

*Cofused
Times*

Health authorities in the post-1974 period were, as now, expected to respond to whatever the latest ministerial passion happened to be. As a consequence, the NHS's mission and purpose has always been somewhat muddled and seemingly all things to all men and women. Far from the NHS having a clear sense of strategy at this global level, it remains adrift strategically and this is no less true of the 1970s and 1980s than it is of the 1990s.

The position remains largely unchanged in the mid-1990s. Indeed, the absence of clearly articulated principles has been a particular source of anxiety in respect of the 1991 changes. As a group of policy analysts observed in their commentary on the 1989 White Paper, *Working for Patients*:

Criticism

> 'Principles are an essential prerequisite to service development because they give everyone involved in their development a vision coupled with a real sense of purpose and direction. The White Paper makes no mention of how its reforms will either contribute to or, as many fear, detract from the guiding principles of the NHS, while having plenty to say about specific services. There is no framework to drive the reforms, no benchmark against which to measure their success or failure, and no apparent concern with outcome or impact.' (Harrison *et al.* 1989, p. 12)

*Goal of
74 Reform*

With the introduction for the first time of a formal corporate management structure, the 1974 reorganization 'was intended to have a profound and fundamental effect upon the decision making underpinning the development and delivery of health care services' (Rathwell 1987; p. 1). Indeed, the determination to instil a planning culture into the health service was a key thrust for change. The corporate management structure was designed to bring order to a fragmented NHS just as the formal planning system was intended to introduce some direction to a service which had survived by 'muddling through'.

The new arrangements had their critics on the grounds that the reforms were overly cumbersome, bureaucratic and belonged to an outmoded rationalist tradition best represented by Taylorism and the school of scientific management which was not seen to be appropriate for the NHS. Failure was therefore virtually guaranteed. Barnard (1977) gives four reasons in support of his belief that the 1974 reorganization was destined to fail:

Criticism

- ◆ There is no single product or range of products in the health service which allow rationalization in the interests of efficiency.
- ◆ Consumer behaviour is difficult to understand in the health care context.
- ◆ Conflicting local interests make consultation and collaboration laborious.
- ◆ The dominant feature of health care delivery is one which involves concentrating on relieving present problems and not on the provision or attainment of a desirable state of affairs some time in the future; i.e. the urgent forever drives out the important.

Reasons for failure.

Rathwell (1987) concludes his study of strategic planning in the NHS by cataloguing the reasons for its failure. Chief among these was the separation between management and planning. There was a failure to connect the two. As a consequence, planning was viewed as a highly prescriptive function not keyed into the real world, and management was in practice little more than administration. Rathwell points to **strategic management** as a unifying concept which seeks to bring together planning and management. Strategic management also seeks to combine the discipline of the planning and management function with the flexibility necessary for the development and implementation of policies. Strategic management does not attempt to provide a prescription for problem solving. Rather it seeks to combine the deliberate and the emergent approaches to strategic development considered in the first section of this chapter.

It was mounting frustration over the apparent inability of the elaborate planning system that had been developed through the late 1970s that resulted in the 1980s becoming the decade when politicians struggled through various reform moves to reorient the NHS towards a leaner and more focused management system that would achieve greater output for a given resource. *The theme of the decade was value-for-money and the search for cost improvements.*

As the 1980s progressed, and as the doctrines of the political right got a tighter grip on virtually every policy sector in Britain, there was a growing perception that introducing competitive principles into the NHS, combined with an injection of business management practices, would provide the solution which politicians had long looked for in respect of solving some deep-seated problems in the NHS. At least, that is how the reforms were presented in the 1989 White Paper, *Working for Patients* (Cm 555, 1989).

Prior to the NHS reforms announced in the 1989 White Paper, the NHS had only begun to emerge from a major management restructuring. The introduction of general management in 1982, which followed an inquiry into the management of the NHS chaired by an industrialist, Roy Griffiths, was heralded as the most important change in the culture of the Service (Griffiths 1983). A seasoned NHS administrator/manager has written (Edwards 1993, p. 83):

Aim of Griffiths.

> 'The Griffiths report was not really about managerial structures and arrangements. It was about creating a new energetic, more thrusting and committed style of management ... Griffiths was about creating a culture in which responsibility was pushed down the line as far was possible.'

The quest for improved management, a pertinent feature of successive NHS reorganizations, is relevant to the discussion of strategy because part of the critique of management was the absence of a clear strategy, particularly in respect of central government's responsibilities in this area. The Griffiths report expressed concern over the way in which the centre became involved in the detailed affairs of the Service which suffered from too many fussy directives on operational matters and too little clear direction on overall strategy. If the NHS was guilty of being over-administered and under-managed, as a former Secretary of State for Health alleged, then the government was largely responsible for such a state of affairs.

Health strategy, 1989–1994

The 'business society' ethic which became entrenched in the NHS as a result of implementing the Griffiths recommendations underpinned the thrust of the 1989 reforms, later embraced in the **NHS and Community Care Act 1990** and implemented in April 1991. There was no let up in the 'cult of managerialism' either in the NHS or elsewhere in the public sector. Indeed, the arrival of general management and components of the 1989 reforms, notably the purchaser–provider separation, gave it a renewed impetus known as **New Public Management (NPM)** (Hood 1991). Its principal components are set out in Box 2.1.

NPM is in large measure a reaction to the perceived failure of what might be called old public management or a traditional public administration approach to public sector management. It represents the outcome of the search for different management models noted earlier which was fuelled by a loss of faith in comprehensive,

Box 2.1
Principal doctrines of
new public
management

- ♦ Explicit standards and measures of performance
- ♦ Greater emphasis on outputs, stressing results
- ♦ Disaggregation of public bureaucracies into agencies operating on a user-pay basis
- ♦ Greater competition through use of quasi-markets and contracting
- ♦ Stress on private sector styles of management practice
- ♦ Management style which emphasizes output targets, short-term contracts, monetary incentives
- ♦ Stress on discipline in resource use, cost cutting, cost improvements

Source: Hood (1991)

or synoptic, rational planning led from central government. In contrast, NPM derives its strength from its bottom-up focus on results, on satisfying user preferences, and on quality. In doing so, it reinforces, and gives a sharper edge to, the already existing tension in the NHS between national strategy on the one hand and local strategy on the other. It also contributes to what remains a fundamental strategic contradiction at the heart of the NHS reforms, namely, the purpose of the NHS itself. Does it exist to pursue the collective needs of a community or population, or to meet a series of individually expressed needs and preferences? The reforms, with their basis in competitive market principles and the rhetoric of choice, have created considerable confusion around this issue which remains to be clarified. To compound the confusion, the Secretary of State for Health has restated the key objectives of the NHS as being (DoH 1993a, p. 5):

- ♦ to lead the drive for improvement in the health of the nation;
- ♦ to provide a health service for all, on the basis of clinical need, regardless of ability to pay;
- ♦ to secure continuous improvement in the quality of patient care;
- ♦ to ensure that treatment and care are targeted to meet local needs;
- ♦ to use available resources as efficiently as possible to meet the rising demands and expectations of the public.

Although the care in the community reforms, also announced in 1989, followed a broadly similar prescription to the NHS reforms there is a crucial difference. It concerns the commitment to planning of which there was no mention in the NHS reforms.

Annual community care plans are required, preferably single plans produced jointly by local authority social services departments and health authorities with input as appropriate from the independent sector.

The purchaser–provider separation in health and social care is based on the twin notions of the internal market and managed competition for which the American economist, Alain Enthoven, is chiefly responsible (Enthoven 1985). The assumption is that such an arrangement will improve efficiency and lead to greater responsiveness to users. Essential in the construction of an internal market is the separation of two previously conflated functions: the *provision* of health services, and the *purchase* (or commissioning) of care. The latter function entails the allocation of funds to providing institutions so as to ensure that the needs of a population are met. It was not at first acknowledged that the reforms contained the potential for a new vision of health care. Perhaps this was because the architects of the changes were themselves either unclear as to their purpose or only interested in particular themes. Since the reforms were announced, there have so far been three Secretaries of State for Health and each has pursued a rather different set of principles. *If a coherent vision has always been a key part of the reforms then it has either remained buried or amounts to a post hoc rationalization or piecing together of different strands many of them only loosely connected to the reform proposals.* Part of the Functions and Manpower Review, referred to earlier, is about addressing this issue as it affects strategy formulation at the centre. Setting the strategic direction is seen as the task of central management of the NHS. The strategic framework will include (DoH 1993a, p. 14):

Strategy

- a statement of the results to be achieved by the NHS;
- a strategic view of how services might be shaped and resources used to deliver the intended outcomes;
- derived from this, individual strategies for the main professional and functional areas including public health, nursing, education, finance, human resources and information; and
- a management strategy which integrates the individual professional and functional strategies in a way that ensures they complement rather than conflict with each other.

On top of all this are two related strategic developments which began to shift attention from narrow health care considerations to the complex issue of health. The notion of health gain entered the vocabulary at the time of the reforms, having been blooded in Wales as part of the Welsh Office's efforts to ensure that strategic considerations drive the NHS reforms and not vice versa. The issue of health gain is taken up again in the next section, but it arose in England in the context of the health strategy, *The Health of the*

Nation (Cm 1986, 1992), and the NHS Research and Development strategy, announced in 1991 (DoH 1991, 1993b).

Both these developments are seen as important in providing guiding lights to fledgling purchasers struggling to make sense of their new role, and one for which they feel largely unprepared. The health strategy is seen as providing a welcome framework within which local purchasers can develop local strategies and targets. *The Health of the Nation* identifies five key target areas but also emphasizes the irrelevance of the NHS acting alone in attempting to meet them. An intersectoral approach, particularly involving local government, is essential. While the NHS has an important contribution to make to improving health it is only a contribution and not the total answer. A more holistic view of health and its determinants has begun to surface, although it creates a major problem for purchasers who find it less straightforward to grasp the issues in respect of improving health as distinct from health care. However, it has served to open up new horizons and to stimulate innovative thinking on how health could be improved.

R+D Based ↑

The R&D strategy, announced in 1991, is viewed as important because it is the first the NHS has had. Decision-making tends to be based on hunch, gut feel, or appeasing vested interests. Rarely, if ever, is it based on what does and does not work in medicine. The R&D strategy seeks to facilitate the development of a knowledge-based NHS by making available to managers the results of research both extant and in progress. Research is therefore essential to any strategy to improve health (DoH 1993b). As the Secretary of State for Health stated in a speech delivered at a BMA Conference on priority-setting in May 1993:

> 'Before we can be confident that we are using resources appropriately, we need to have a much better knowledge of the outcomes of clinical interventions. Previously common treatments have been demonstrated to be either ineffective or over-used – for example, grommets or tonsillectomies. At the same time, we need to understand more clearly the health gain that can be obtained from different procedures – for example, hip replacements or medical treatments for leukaemia.'

Both the health and R&D strategies are centrally led initiatives but each has a local dimension in order to appear relevant to local circumstances and to secure effective implementation. This is important because unless new ways of thinking about health and about R&D enter into the organizational bloodstream at local level, they will fail in their endeavours. These issues are as important for the NHS trusts as they are for purchasers. Trusts must also produce strategies in the form of an annual business plan if they are to develop and survive. They cannot rely on the *status quo* remaining intact even if this is the wish of many of them.

It can be deduced from the above that neither purchasers nor providers have found creating health strategy an easy task. For some it seems either a luxury or a cruel diversion from the pressures of surviving each day as it comes. For others, the financial pressures to deliver a balanced budget eclipse all other considerations however intrinsically desirable they may be. Finally, the reforms themselves have some way still to run and a period of stability, or freezing, seems a long way off if it ever arises. Managers and others are having to become accustomed to continual change. While this may contribute to the importance strategy *should* have in helping to guide the change, it also diverts attention from strategic considerations in an effort to respond to, and sort out, the latest crisis or directive from above.

Having considered the overall background to, and context of, the reforms, it is time to move on and examine how purchasers and providers respectively are going about the task of creating health strategies in the early years of the changes.

HEALTH STRATEGY: THE PURCHASER ROLE

There are three NHS purchasing agencies: district health authorities, FHSAs and GPFHs, the latter also being providers. Since late 1993, DHAs and FHSAs are being encouraged to merge although legislation will not be passed to allow this before 1996.

The strategy formulation role of purchasing authorities is simple enough to state though complex to execute. *In essence it is to purchase services which will enhance the health of populations and local communities having first defined what the need of those populations and communities are.* The role of purchasers is seen as critical in shaping the strategic direction of health and health care policy and practice. The enormity of the challenge is at odds with the belated attention given to the purchasing role. For the first couple of years of the reforms purchasing was virtually ignored as the government devoted its attention to trusts and GP fundholders. As a result, purchasing at DHA level got off to a slow start and lost senior management talent to the more lucrative and powerful trusts. Most managers, trained as providers, felt more affinity with the provider role and were uncertain of what a purchasing role would entail in practice. The government in 1993 decided that purchasing should be at the top of the health service agenda. A purchaser-driven NHS is now the goal and its five key elements are set out in Box 2.2.

Emphasis on Purchasers.

The concept of health gain is crucial to the strategic role of purchasing agencies. The reason this is important is that, although the term lacks precise meaning, it embraces a number of issues and initiatives, including developments in needs assessment, health outcomes, listening to local people, and health services research, which are seen as central elements of a health strategy. Defining and agreeing what constitutes effective health care or good

Box 2.2
Key elements of a
purchaser-driven NHS

◆ Purchasing must reach out to the future, not simply repli-
cate the past; it will involve a shift away from the status
quo

◆ An element of competition between providers, and also
between purchasers is vital for change

◆ There must be shared purchasing between health
authorities and all GPs (including fundholders); all family
doctors must be closely involved in the purchasing process

◆ Contracting between purchasers and providers is a
powerful mechanism for change, but it needs development. Doctors and nurses must become more closely
involved in the contracting process

◆ Purchasing is about developing and managing relationships. Its successful development will require effective
leadership and commitment.

Source: Mawhinney and Nichol (1993)

performance or a successful outcome is not straightforward. In the
past, health planning has focused on *structure* (or inputs) and on
process (or outputs). Only since the 1991 reforms has attention
turned to outcomes. Health gain is concerned with improving
health status which means the production of positive outcomes.
But the matter of outcomes is complex and purchasers are only just
beginning to consider how they can best be incorporated in their
decision-making. Health authorities, for the most part, are still at
the stage of comprehending the precise nature of their strategic
role in the context of health gain. Effective purchasing is seen as
taking a strategic approach to delivering demonstrable improvements in people's health. As the former Minister for Health, Brian
Mawhinney, put it in one of three keynote speeches setting out the
challenge for purchasers:

> [Health authorities] 'need to think beyond the annual purchasing
> cycle and take at least a five-year forward look, within the context of
> national and regional priorities. They should adopt a "no surprises"
> policy. For example, they need to give providers some idea about
> long-term purchasing intentions to enable them to prepare capital
> investment plans. Equally, though, purchasers need to be clear what
> they are trying to achieve themselves. Their strategy should contain
> clear health targets and identify how progress towards them is going
> to be measured.' (Mawhinney and Nichol 1993, p. 17)

For Dr Mawhinney, *strategy* constitutes the first of his seven
main 'stepping stones' to successful purchasing (see Box 2.3). In
fact most, if not all, of the seven steps are important in respect of

Box 2.3
Seven stepping stones
for effective purchasing

♦ a strategic view

♦ robust contracts

♦ knowledge-based decisions

♦ responsiveness to local people

♦ mature relations with providers

♦ local alliances

♦ organizational fitness

Source: Mawhinney and Nichol (1993, p. 21)

strategy formulation and its subsequent implementation. For instance, purchasing decisions should be *knowledge-based* rather than, as all too often occurred in the past, based on hunch and intuition. Decisions are expected to be 'based on sound evidence about health needs, clinical and cost-effectiveness, and costs and prices' (*ibid*. p. 18). To this end, the R&D strategy is seen as having a critical role. Introduced in 1991, the strategy, and accompanying infrastructure, is intended to promote applied research that is of relevance to the delivery of health care services and to shift the balance from biomedical research to health services research. A key challenge facing the R&D strategy is to provide evidence on what works and does not work in medicine and then to assist in the process of using that knowledge to change behaviour and practice. As a prerequisite, it is necessary to create a research culture within NHS management where traditionally decisions have been taken for reasons that have less to do with knowledge about effectiveness and more to do with history, professional power, organizational inertia and media attention.

Necessity

Responsiveness to local people is seen as important because strategy formulation is not regarded as the exclusive preserve of professionals determining what is important. Improving people's health must mean involving public and patients in that process. Most health authorities have gone far in involving Community Health Councils in strategy development but rather fewer have sought other ways of engaging with the public. Experiments have occurred with public or consumer surveys aimed at identifying need but also at collecting views about priorities. By April 1994 every health authority was required to demonstrate that it was seriously seeking and acting on the views of the public and its representatives.

Positive + Negative

The issue of involving the public in strategy is linked to the sensitive matter of *rationing and priority-setting*. Up until the

Rationing

Criticism

reforms, rationing remained largely invisible and implicit with decisions about access to care made by clinicians ostensibly on medical grounds. The purchaser–provider split has resulted in greater explicitness as purchasers, through the contracting mechanism, must state what they will purchase and, therefore, what they will not. This has raised concerns about the legitimacy of appointed bodies to take decisions that are not technical in context but are essentially political, involving the exercise of values and judgement. Many managers in particular feel uncomfortable at making choices like, for instance, whether to purchase IVF services, and one reason for seeking the public's views is to obtain an idea of the community's views when it comes to priority-setting and making choices. What remains unclear is how the information gathered from public consultation exercises of various kinds is actually incorporated into the judgements and decisions of health authorities. Moreover, a public debate about rationing is difficult when the scope for redeploying resources from ineffective procedures and practices to more effective ones is considerable (Hunter 1993b).

Need For competition + co op

Relations with providers are regarded as vital. The term 'mature' has been applied to these in recognition of the tendency, especially early on in the reforms, to adopt inappropriate macho behaviour with the purchaser–provider split being interpreted to mean a 'stand-off' adversarial relationship between purchasers and providers. The Minister for Health accepts the need for 'a creative tension and robust negotiation' between the two parties but at the same time stresses the need for partnerships and long-term agreements akin to market relationships in the private sector. Essentially there are two purchasing paradigms: (a) independence and self-interest, and (b) interdependence and mutuality. The characteristics of each are listed in Box 2.4.

Alliances To Promote Health

Finally, the creation and maintenance of *local alliances* is an important part of strategy, especially in the context of the health strategy with its acknowledgement of the key role played by non-NHS agencies, notably local government. The NHS's contribution to improving health, as distinct from alleviating pain and suffering, is limited. Other agencies have as much or more to contribute. Hence the jargon term 'healthy alliances'. The attempt to build local alliances has led to efforts to introduce joint commissioning arrangements across health and local authorities although these are not yet common. A major obstacle to creating local alliances is the different cultures, priorities and ways of working to be found in health and local authorities. Nevertheless, proposals have been put forward for integrated health and social welfare agencies (Health Services Management Unit 1992) or for putting the health purchasing function with local government (Harrison *et al.* 1991). *The Health of the Nation*, doubtless unintentionally, lends some support to this option. It states (paras 3.11 and 3.13):

Box 2.4
Purchasing mindsets

Paradigm 1	Paradigm 2
Independent Interest	*Mutuality of Interest*
◆ 'I Win'	◆ 'I Win You Win'
◆ Demand All, Give Nothing	◆ Shared Risks
◆ Commercially Aggressive	◆ Commercially Assertive, Not Cosy
◆ 'Supplier Problems Are Their Problems'	◆ Developing Supplier Capabilities
	◆ Partnerships
Profit Maximization	*Success Maximization*
◆ Short Term	◆ Long Term
◆ Price, Cost Critical	◆ Robust Value Chain
◆ Sealed Bids, Dutch Auctions	◆ Emphasis on Value
Uninhibited Competition	*Restrained Competition*
◆ Dog Eat Dog, Capricious	◆ Appropriate Stability
◆ More Competition is Best	◆ Appropriate Competition
Information for Power	*Information for Joint Action*
◆ Information to Punish	◆ Joint Problem-Solving

Source: Trent RHA (1992)

'[Local authorities] are responsible for protecting the environment in which people live and work. They are also responsible for the purchasing and direct provision of social services to meet the needs of individual members of the public who live in their area. Environmental health departments have a special part to play with their responsibilities for health and safety at work, for food safety and food quality, and in collaboration with health authorities for health promotion and investigating and bringing under control outbreaks of communicable disease. . . . [Any] of these responsibilities on their own would make the input of local authorities to the strategy for health significant. Taken together the contribution of local authorities is vital.'

welsh example.

Of course, to deliver on the new and evolving purchasing agenda requires organizational capacity, a topic considered in the final section of this chapter.

Within the UK, the Welsh have gone furthest in developing a strategic approach in the pursuit of health gain at the national (i.e. all Wales) and local levels. Developed by the Welsh Health Planning

Forum, *Strategic Intent and Direction for the NHS in Wales* is the vehicle for taking the people of Wales into the 21st century. Precisely because the pace of change is so rapid in health and social care, good strategic planning is deemed essential. 'All organisations need a strategy' (Welsh Health Planning Forum 1989a, para 2, 9). Strategic direction should be focused on health gain, centred on people and effective in the use of resources.

The approach argues that in the past strategy has been driven by provider-related issues, particularly manpower, building and equipment. It has served to distract managers and clinicians from the underlying purpose of the NHS which is to secure better health for the population as a whole. The Welsh approach is shown in Figure 2.2. It regards strategic planning as a way of 'becoming more focused on the future' (*ibid.*, para 12, 13). However, it acknowledges that 'strategic plans often reveal more about today's problems than tomorrow's opportunities. With the introduction of new technologies, medical advances, and other uncertainties, the predictive horizon is becoming shorter'. The Welsh approach to strategic planning is a structured process linking the three phases of direction, formulation and implementation.

Progress is not, generally speaking, as well advanced in England although some RHAs are adopting a similar approach with their purchaser agencies. Trent Health is one example with its *Strategy of Health*, derived from WHO *Health for All* principles, which is based on the work of Joint Purchasing Executives between DHAs, FHSAs and GPs (see subsection below on joint commissioning). The Trent Strategy is being taken forward through a Health Gain Investment Programme (see Box 2.5).

Joint commissioning With the separation of purchasing between DHAs, FHSAs and GPFHs it was quickly acknowledged by some Regions, and by the Department of Health/NHSE, that such an arrangement would make it more difficult to coordinate commissioning in a way that furthered policy in the direction of achieving effective links, and an integrated strategy, across primary and secondary care. Moreover, unless some type of **joint commissioning** was put in place, the split budget between primary and secondary care would make it all but impossible to achieve any strategic shift between these sectors.

The first step in joint commissioning is to secure common boundaries between DHAs and FHSAs. Joint commissioning is designed to facilitate alliances with voluntary and community groups that are vital to health promotion and care in the community. Links with local government are seen as especially important for reasons noted earlier – principally its contribution to the *Health of the Nation* agenda. Joint commissioning also reaffirms primary care as being at the centre of health care services – not the restricted notion of primary health care with which we are all familiar but a broad conception of primary health which, in

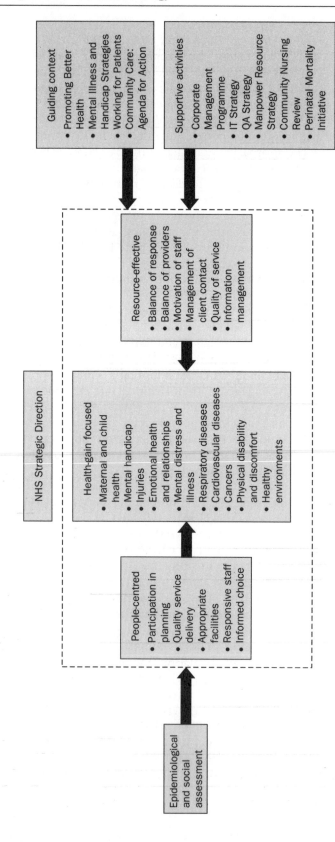

Figure 2.2
Strategic direction: the NHS in Wales
Source: Welsh Health Planning Forum 1989a, p. 25)

Box 2.5
Trent RHA health
gain investment
programme

The Health Gain Investment Programme (HGIP) has been developed within eight programme areas shown to bring about the greatest health gain:

♦ cardiovascular disease
♦ pregnancy and childbirth
♦ diabetes
♦ infant and child health
♦ mental health
♦ lung cancer
♦ HIV/AIDS
♦ disability

Each programme consists of an exercise in health policy analysis, setting known information about the effectiveness, efficiency, appropriateness and acceptability of available service options against the background of relevant epidemiology.

To complement HGIP a series of Focus Guides is being produced, providing information on good practice in service delivery and the organization of services. The guides are intended to assist purchasers in drawing up service specifications and agreeing standards.

addition to the usual range of services, includes community health services, primary care by accident and emergency departments, outpatient and day care services by hospitals, a list of secondary care services transferable to primary care providers, self-referral services by patients, and social care.

Joint commissioning aims at 'seamless care', based on need, by the most appropriate and cost-effective providers working with clear protocols and good measures of health gain from a single cash pool to facilitate resource transfers between secondary and primary care. Such a model demands a lot of GPs, possibly more than many can, or are prepared to, offer. GPs will cease to be independent contractors and become managers of primary care services.

In an unpublished study of joint commissioning for North West Thames RHA, Light (1993) describes two approaches to joint commissioning: organic and structural. The *organic approach* focuses on people, on dialogue, joint appointments, on forging common value sets and agendas, and on developing joint projects. In contrast, the *structural approach* focuses on getting the organizational and management arrangements right. Most changes in the NHS follow the latter approach, which may not be the most successful or sustainable. Both approaches depend on strong, stable leadership – a scarce commodity in the NHS at the present time when the turnover rate among senior managers is exceptionally high, the average length of time in a top post being just over two years.

In his review of joint commissioning, Light identifies a number of obstacles to its realization:

- contradictions, and lack of coherence, in national policy;
- lack of integrated budgets;
- professional balkanization as different groups claim territory for themselves;
- GPFH emphasizes independence not cooperation or team playing;
- differences in language, culture, priorities and organization between DHAs, FHSAs, GPs, consultants and trusts;
- different ways of costing and pricing services;
- lack of strong leadership;
- lack of community understanding and support;
- lack of consumer information about services and options.

Light regards joint commissioning as inevitable and desirable if the contradictions between needs-based purchasing by DHAs and fundholding by GPs, with its attendant risks of fragmentation, are to be successfully tackled. The government's decision to encourage, though not require, mergers between DHAs and FHSAs recognizes the importance of the issue.

Joint commissioning does two things:

Perhaps This Marks The Way Forward

- It puts primary care at the centre of the NHS, which has been dominated since its inception by hospitals and capital developments.
- It represents a fundamental shift from managed *competition* to managed *cooperation*.

In addition, a single health commission facilitates the implementation of joint initiatives with local government in the area of community care and in achieving the targets set out in the health strategy which, we may recall from the earlier discussion, require local authority input.

Contracts

Pragmatism By Cons

The mechanism whereby purchasers' strategic intentions are translated into practice is the contract. Contracting for health care is a new activity in the British NHS and the process is very much one of 'learning by doing'. To date, a pragmatic approach has been adopted whereby contracting has been subject to a tightly managed approach in order not to destabilize existing services or to trigger abrupt changes.

Takes Up Time.

NHS contracts are not legally binding documents and in practice resemble service agreements. Most contracts are negotiated and placed annually, a practice which has led to what is known as the 'contracting treadmill' whereby for two or three months each year health care managers are preoccupied with contract negotiations thus distracting them from other matters. There are moves to place contracts for two to three years at a stretch and to ensure that these are monitored on a regular ongoing basis rather than annually.

There are two principal types of contract being operated by health care purchasers (see Box 2.6 for details):

♦ **cost-per-case contracts;**
♦ **block contracts.**

A particular issue that arises in the context of GP fundholders is that high **transaction costs** may be involved, with providers sometimes negotiating with a large number of purchasers in the shape of GP fundholders. The long-term effects of this problem as more fundholders become established have not been estimated but it is an issue that requires close monitoring.

In general, contracting has not been used to alter the present configuration of services. Purchasers, for the most part, remain weak and at the mercy of providers who all too often decide what they are going to do and then look to the purchaser to pay. Purchasers are invariably confronted by a *fait accompli* in the absence of evidence to hand that a procedure is ineffective. Even if effective, an intervention like cochlear implants may only be effective for a particular target group. For other people it may be less effective or ineffective, but providers will press to have the threshold lowered to allow access to more patients, therefore driving up costs. Adverse media coverage along the lines of a child being denied treatment and other examples of 'shroud waving' make purchasers nervous about challenging providers' decisions.

Yet, if purchasing is to succeed and is to drive the agenda then provider preferences cannot be allowed to determine the type and amount of services provided. If they are, then the role of purchasers becomes largely redundant. The dilemma gives added impetus to the R&D strategy and to the need for this to deliver in respect of good evaluative evidence and health technology assessment. At the same time, managers are looking to their public health colleagues to collect and use such evidence to inform decision-making (Richardson, Duggan and Hunter 1994). Initiatives like the Effective Health Care bulletins, the UK Clearing House on Health Outcomes Assessment and the Review and Dissemination Centre are all usefully providing purchasers with ammunition to use in negotiations with providers but their impact remains unknown.

GPs and purchasing   For GPs, the NHS reforms have resulted in significant implications for the way they operate particularly if they have acquired fundholding status. The government is committed to extending GP fundholding in order to encourage a primary care-led NHS in which GPs progressively become the principal purchasers for a range of services (NHS Executive 1994). As fundholders, GPs are both purchasers and providers. Fundholding GPs have a budget with which to buy drugs and appliances, paramedical services,

Box 2.6
Types of contracts

Cost-per-case contracts
In this form of contract, a cost or price is set for each type of treatment that is delivered. Contract prices can be set on an **average cost basis** or on a **marginal cost basis** where there is excess capacity in the system. In the current British NHS, there is very little excess capacity which makes this form of contracting unpopular. In cost-per-case contracts, prices are regulated so that NHS trusts are required to make a 6% return on their assets each year.

Cost-per-case contracts require a greater degree of price information than is currently available in the NHS where information systems remain variable and in some cases quite poor. In most cases individual treatment costs are not known with any degree of precision. The database can be expected to improve over the next few years and there are already moves to encourage the development of clinical protocols and their application in respect of contracts.

A further problem with cost-per-case contracts is that they are costly to write (because of the level of information they require), to implement (because of the detail involved in ensuring that they are followed correctly to the letter and not merely to the spirit), and to enforce (sophisticated marketing systems are required). It is no accident, therefore, that only 14% of first-wave trusts back in 1992 intended operating cost-per-case contracts.

Block contracts
The block contract is sometimes known as an incomplete contract in which the purchaser agrees to pay the provider, in this case the NHS trust, an annual fee in return for access to a broadly-defined range of services. The commissioner or purchaser of care will lay down in the contract broad performance targets such as an increase in the proportion of day cases, maximum targets for waiting lists, and reduced lengths of stay. However, these targets are related to process issues rather than outcomes in respect of impact on patients or on care. The block contract will specify how quality is to be monitored and, again, this is an area that is relatively undeveloped in the UK.

The real problem with block contracts is the information asymmetry that exists between the purchaser and provider concerning the level to which the contract is fulfilled. Effective block contracts are heavily reliant upon high trust relationships. In their absence, the contract is open to what is known as 'opportunism'. In such cases, the provider can vary its performance strategy and choose a set of actions which may not optimize the purchaser's interests but will certainly seek to optimize the provider's. This means that the level of service that is delivered according to the contract could be at too high a level or could be at too low a level. This could, in turn, result in an overall increase in the cost of service delivery over and above that which might have obtained under the previous pre-1991 integrated planning and delivery service.

Block contracts therefore carry a high degree of risk for the provider. This is because the purchaser will preset the volume of work to be undertaken and pay for this accordingly but it will not always be possible for the provider to know in advance the various conditions and influences that might affect his ability to deliver on that contract. Quite often, circumstances beyond his control can arise and serve to increase the costs that he will incur in providing that level of service. So, where the contract fee is fixed in advance but the delivery costs in practice are variable, the provider is liable to carry the risk unless there is some attempt at risk sharing between purchaser and provider. Certainly, the risk factor will increase the costs of operating a block contract system.

There is a third form of contract – **cost and volume contracts** – but it is essentially a mix of the other two.

some hospital services and community health services. They are free to negotiate their own contracts with individual providers and shop around to get the best value for money on behalf of their patients. Fundholding has both positive and negative features (Pietroni 1993). Among the former are:

◆ the opportunity and freedom to make decisions about where contracts are placed;
◆ greater access to hospital services and enhanced freedom of referral; and
◆ the possibility of making savings through prudent management which can be invested in other aspects of the practice.

From the limited research undertaken on **GPFH**, the work by Glennerster and his colleagues (1994) concludes that GPFH is a success story of the reforms as it has put the patient first and has effectively challenged the monopoly power of hospital consultants. Instead of planning being a top-down process, GPFH has resulted in empowering patients. It has shifted the balance of power and finance from the top of the service to the bottom. It puts purchasing power and choice nearer the patient, informed by his or her doctor (*ibid.*).

Other commentators, like Pietroni (1993), remain more sceptical and point to the many disadvantages of the scheme. As the budget for GPFH practices is taken out of a district's total allocation, fragmentation is the result as the district's purchasing power, and scope for achieving strategic change, is reduced. This may, in turn, reduce the district's ability to develop suitable contracts for all patients with the result that a two-tier system is the inevitable consequence. *GPFHs possess the means, therefore, whereby they may, if unintentionally, distort the priorities for care set by the health authority.* A district with several GPFH practices could easily find its strategic plan significantly affected. GPFH places new obligations upon GPs in respect of improved information and management systems. However, patients may wonder if decisions are based on clinical need or on financial considerations.

GPs ought to be the main beneficiaries of the strategic shift from secondary to primary care but many view it with considerable suspicion and cynicism. They do not believe that appropriate investment in primary care will occur and consider that they will continue to be a dumping ground for patients and society's rejects unable to get hospital treatment or be treated elsewhere.

Extra-contractual referrals (ECRs) pose another problem and are a source of growing unease between GPs and health authorities. In most areas, the ECR budget has been overspent and attempts are being made to encourage GPs not to use ECRs indiscriminately or to get faster treatment for patients. But if GPs' freedom of referral is sacrosanct it is not possible to go further unless, as is happening in some places, health authorities refuse to sanction ECRs. GPs are an important group who cannot be left out of the commissioning process. In many districts collaborative arrangements are in place and GPs are organizing themselves into appropriate groups so as to impact on the commissioning process. So, there has been a move from competition, spurred on by GPFH, to collaboration. *GPs will at this strategic level become involved in setting priorities even if some are sceptical about doing so because of the time involved and because of a fear that it will erode their traditional, and much cherished, independence.*

Care in the community

The community care reforms, implemented over a three-year period between 1991 and 1993, are similarly committed to a strategic approach. Indeed, in contrast to the NHS reforms, the term 'planning' has not been abandoned in the 1989 White Paper, *Caring for People* (Cm 849). There is much emphasis on the need for local authorities to produce community care plans, preferably jointly with health authorities. As in the NHS, social services departments are expected to develop a purchaser–provider separation, form collaborative links with other agencies, and involve users at the various stages of the process.

The development of a mixed economy of care is proceeding cautiously and at a slower pace than the NHS changes. In a study of 24 Social Service Departments (SSDs) aimed at exploring the initial steps taken to prepare for the new enabling role, Wistow *et al.* (1992) found, perhaps predictably, that few authorities had drawn up precise plans for the purchaser–provider split. Only two had achieved some degree of split. The rest were either opposed to it or more lukewarm or non-committal. The researchers also found few authorities prepared actively to encourage independent sector providers.

The emphasis on **pluralism** in the community care reforms poses problems while also ensuring jointness and partnership among providers and agencies, which is the point of joint plans between SSDs and health authorities. As lead agencies for community care, SSDs need to ensure the commitment of health authorities and a range of providers, including the independent sector, to the changes. This is particularly problematic with respect to the NHS preoccupied as it is with its own reforms.

The development of a market and competition in social care is constrained, not only by professional and/or organizational factors, but also by the existence of other factors. Wistow *et al.* (1992) identify four:

♦ *too few suppliers* – which makes moving away from direct monopoly provision virtually impossible;
♦ *the sloping playing field* –which queers the pitch for SSDs who believe the independent sector is being granted an unfair advantage over them;
♦ *high transaction costs* and the contract culture is demanding in terms of ensuring quality and appropriate outcomes;

♦ *price or quality competition* – there was a widespread belief among SSDs in the study that a classic market situation would not be possible and that abuses would occur and choice for users would prove to be illusory.

Wistow *et al.* conclude that 'these concerns about market forces underlie the present reluctance of most authorities to develop social care markets'.

An Audit Commission assessment of the community care reforms some six months into their implementation concludes that 'cautious but steady progress has been made' while conceding that 'for the full benefit to be realised a wider range of options for care must be developed' (Audit Commission 1993, p. 1.). Certainly the chaos predicted after 1 April 1993 has not occurred. Nevertheless, as an SSI/RHA monitoring exercise demonstrates, medium and longer term strategy development is a priority (DoH 1993c). In particular, the strategic shift under way in the health care sector will have a major impact on local authority SSDs. Community care planning is seen as the mechanism for close working between health and local authorities.

Another interim assessment found that while 'a steady hold on the system has been maintained', *users, carers and their advocates see little or no improvement in the system and in services* (Robinson and Wistow 1993). In some ways they are worse off, with access to free health care being replaced by social services for which a charge is made. The development and promotion of joint commissioning of community care is advocated in order to pool resources to tackle problems on the health and social care boundary.

HEALTH STRATEGY: THE PROVIDER ROLE

Strategy development in the provider units, over 90% of which have been trusts since April 1994, is as varied and problematic as it is for purchasers. Many hospital and community health trusts have focused on operational rather than strategic planning. They have been more concerned about survival and at succeeding in winning contracts than about the strategic direction they may wish to take in future. Moreover, there are often difficult relations with purchasers which makes it all too easy for providers to produce their own plans in complete isolation from purchasers who may have different ideas about what to buy. There are major issues involved which require for their effective resolution close relations between purchasers and providers.

For most providers, the annual contracting round and the evolving internal market are the twin issues which are occupying them. Concern centres on whether they are deemed preferred providers or whether competition is to be encouraged by purchasers. In other words, when relations are cosy there is less onus on providers to look strategically at what they have to offer.

Capital development under trusts has changed little from the arrangements in existence before the reforms despite the fact that promised freedoms over capital were one of the chief attractions of trust status. The bulk of capital funds are allocated through a project approval process operated until April 1994 by seven outposts of the NHSME. Under the new arrangement of eight Regional Offices, the monitoring function in respect of purchasers and providers is combined in the one organization (DoH 1993a).

The main strategic issues affecting providers include the medical revolution under way in respect of new treatments and less invasive surgery which question the present location, configuration and size of hospitals whose pattern stems from the 1962 Hospital Plan. The rapid changes in the delivery of care make the concept of the district general hospital redundant. Coupled with a move towards primary and community care as a means of locating care closer to people's homes, the future of hospitals is a major issue which is under discussion in commissioning agencies across the country if not trusts.

Competitive forces introduced by the 1991 reforms are likely to have two effects, both of which will have a significant impact upon the operation of acute units (Newchurch 1992). Competition will speed up the implementation of productivity and technological change as units seek comparative advantage, and it will expose inefficiencies and overcapacity within the system. For managers of acute hospitals in particular, the strategic dilemma is considerable. So far, they have viewed their role as one of preserving, and if possible expanding, the institution for which they are responsible. That, after all, is the source of pressures within the hospital to which they have sought to respond. A result of this strategy has been that many hospitals have looked for cost-cutting opportunities while trying to retain services along existing lines but with increasingly limited resources. But as Newchurch points out '*attempting to maintain the status quo may ultimately prove disastrous in its failure to address the underlying strategic issues*' (*ibid.*, p. 5).

The key to survival and success for an acute hospital lies in the introduction of dynamic and continuous change focused on five key areas:

◆ skill mix;
◆ configuration;
◆ operational effectiveness;
◆ asset utilization;
◆ management role and function.

Of these, the configuration issue is of particular significance. Traditional configurations are being questioned partly as a result of the desired shift to primary and community care, and partly because of the growing overcapacity of acute units. A redefinition of acute hospitals is under way although it remains at this stage an issue for debate and planning rather than action. The most important consequence of this questioning of the role of the acute hospital is a recognition of the need to decouple the provision of secondary and tertiary acute services from the acute hospital site.

There is a view that the creation of trusts actually makes it more difficult to achieve the strategic shift from secondary to primary care since their very existence serves to strengthen and entrench hospitals. While some trusts may be considering establishing innovative, community based outreach services, none sees its role as one of seriously dismembering the hospital services which it has inherited and on which trust status was granted in the first place. Moreover, given the provider-led initial phase of the reforms and the general weakness of purchasers, hospital trusts have enjoyed a head start in establishing a firm base. An added factor in their favour is the public's emotional attachment to their local hospital and their suspicion of any attempts to rationalize services by shifting to primary care, on the grounds that such a move must mean cuts and inferior services. Hospital closures incite passions which make politicians nervous even if, on occasion, as in London post-Tomlinson, they are prepared to grasp most of the nettle. As Light observes, 'very few failing trusts are allowed to fail' (Light 1993, p. 54). Wresting funds from the hospital sector will therefore be no easy matter. Yet this is the principal source of funds to redirect work towards primary and community care.

There is yet little evidence on how hospital trusts are adapting to significant changes in what might be termed the health care industry. There are a number of practitioner accounts (see, for instance, Part 2 of Tilley, 1993) but no independent systematic research. A further area for development is the mix of public-private provision of health care. The government is keen to promote joint venture arrangements between NHS providers and the private sector as a way of attracting additional resources to the health sector without putting a further burden on the public purse. This area is likely to develop rapidly over the next few years as a consequence of the Private Finance Initiative which requires NHS trusts and purchasers to seek private capital in preference to public funds. The process will need to be carefully and skilfully managed if the NHS is not to be seen as territory ripe for rich pickings by the private health care sector. This is a real danger as the NHS – at all levels – lacks business sector expertise and acumen which might avoid such an outcome. Moreover, blurring the public–private sector boundary raises questions about access and equity which are core principles of the NHS.

AN INTERIM ASSESSMENT: WHITHER STRATEGY?

There are essentially two camps when it comes to an assessment of whether the move to a contract culture in health and social care is likely to lead to provision that reflects need and is sensitive to users' preferences, or whether it is a cynical or dogma-driven exercise designed to do little other than dismantle public sector monopoly provision, regardless of its quality or effectiveness, and cut costs. There are the pessimists and the optimists.

In so much of the government's health sector reform strategy the destination of the various changes – the vision – is either unclear or obscured by a heavy concentration on the chosen means. Indeed, there is a risk of the means becoming the ends, or at any rate substituting for them. Such loose coupling between means and ends risks goal displacement on a grand scale where strategy is neither deliberate nor emergent but simply non-existent. Where the policy ends are not clearly articulated and made explicit then the 'nuts and bolts' management and structural issues obscure, and almost become substitutes for, the emergent policy ends. Two major issues merit attention in this respect.

First, does a market in health and social care facilitate collaborative working across professions and agencies as is required by the emphasis on health gain? Or will it breed suspicion and low trust among the various stakeholders rendering integrated care a forlorn hope and resulting, if by default, in fragmented planning and provision? The ruling by the Ombudsman that Leeds Healthcare failed by not providing long-term care free within the NHS for a brain-damaged stroke victim discharged to a private nursing home because there was nothing more which hospital treatment could do raises key questions nationally about who is responsible for continuing care of chronically ill patients (Health Service Commissioner 1994). Subsequent guidance on the health–social care interface, leaving the matter to be resolved locally, fails to address the problem in the context of a *national* health service. However, it acknowledges that the NHS has a role in continuing care and cannot opt out.

Issues like joint needs assessment, joint commissioning, the sharing of information and care management are all seen as central to the avoidance of fragmented care. Yet, as a result of the market that is developing in health and social care, health authorities are concentrating on what they perceive to be their core business – acute care – and withdrawing from continuing care which is perceived to be the responsibility of social services departments and not the NHS. Unilateral action by health authorities has been criticized by the NHSME and Social Services Inspectorate but, as the Leeds case reported above demonstrates, pressures on budgets and from the marketplace are leading managers anxious to contain spending to raise questions about where health care ends and social care begins. The incentive is to cost shunt cases onto local authority budgets and vice versa. An added complication is that health care remains free while social care is increasingly subject to charging.

It may be that the 'contract culture' will mature and that as managers acquire new skills (still for the most part in their infancy) and confidence and build new relationships acceptable agreements and trade-offs will be negotiated. The problem, and challenge, is that no-one really knows what will happen. The policy and organizational landscape remains unstable and turbulent. To cope, health and social care organizations must become learning organizations prepared and able to adapt flexibly as the market develops (Schon 1973). This is why the concept of *emergent strategy* is so important in a context of rapid and continuous change. But to function in such a way does require having a clear vision of the desired endpoint and one that is effectively communicated, and shared, by all those affected.

A more optimistic scenario suggests that the reforms do provide opportunities to address some long-standing concerns, among them bureaucratic, sclerotic, overlapping, unresponsive services often provided by uncommunicative, uncooperative, insensitive, paternalistic or patronizing professionals.

At the end of the day the reforms will be judged according to the extent to which they yield the benefits promised by their advocates. That is why the strategic dimension is so vital. Evidence from the USA suggests that the operation and practice of contracting in health and social care are fraught with problems. Contracting, as described earlier, is the instrument through which strategy is translated into practice. Smith and Lipsky (1992) argue that 'the model of market competition cannot be used as a means to improve government effectiveness through contracting because in health and social services it is particularly difficult to measure performance'. They maintain that contracting can have advantages but that these should be seen to lie in service needs rather than in the elusive, and possibly illusory, benefits of market competition. This means paying rather less attention to political ideology and rather more to performance assessment and whether contracted out services really are more effective.

A major difficulty with providing any reasoned assessment of the NHS and community care reforms is the absence of reliable research findings coupled with the continuous unfolding of the reforms. As Maynard (1993, p. 66) has concluded 'the reforms are providing advantages and disadvantages and the balance of these effects is unknown'. In the absence of proper systematic evaluation of the reforms it is impossible to determine whether competition in health care is inefficient or whether the overall effect of the changes will result in a net gain when compared with the pre-1991 approach to strategy, planning and management. The evidence from the USA about managed care is similarly absent or incomplete (Miller and Luft 1991). Everywhere, then, competitive mechanisms are advocated but with little empirical support. The few small studies of the British reforms are inevitably inconclusive and incomplete but all agree that it is not yet possible to point to any major changes in strategic direction resulting from them (see chapters in Tilley, 1993, Le Grand and Bartlett 1993, Robinson and Le Grand, 1994). All would probably agree with Maynard that '*the use of market mechanisms in health care systems involves large increases in management costs with as yet unproven benefits in terms of resource allocation*' (*ibid.*, p. 67).

It could be said that competition is unnecessary and will prove to be a less effective and more costly instrument to achieve what ought to be possible through strategic management if there were real commitment to it. The failings of health service planning in the 1970s may have had less to do with the principle and more to do with the approach adopted which ignored the politics of organizational life and neglected the stratagems which need to be deployed to effect change. The advocates of competition cannot so far be said to have grasped these lessons. Certainly the onus is firmly on them to demonstrate that competition is superior in achieving health goals and will not simply result in greater inequities and a reduction in the accessibility of some services. For the House of Commons Social Services Committee, reporting at the time of the White Paper announcing the reforms, a major concern was that an internal market in health care was not good for patients even if it was good for managers and providers (Social Services Committee 1989). Its principal fears about an internal market included the following:

Fears
Int mkt

◆ Patients may have less immediate access to hospital treatment if they have to travel far for specialized treatment.
◆ There are potential financial and other difficulties for patients having to travel longer distances for treatment.
◆ There would be considerable cost consequences of going over to a system of trading in health services.

The Committee expressed further concerns over the difficulty of operating an effective internal market in the absence of accurate data for the costing of treatments and other procedures. It felt that aspects of the market such as GPFHs competing with DHAs as purchasers of care would give rise to the potential for considerable 'gaming'. Other issues remained to be fully worked out, including:

◆ how services could be better planned;
◆ how access to care could be guaranteed and patient choice extended; and
◆ the monitoring and regulation of the quality of services.

Three years after the start of the implementation process it remains the case that the Committee's concerns are for the most part still valid.

Why
Co-op

What has become clear is the need for purchasers and providers to adopt a *modus vivendi* based on mutuality (see paradigm 2, Box 2.4). If purchasing for the health care needs of the population in the 21st century is going to mean putting a brake on the capital programme so that it is realigned with the policy thrust in favour of developing primary and community care, then providers must be central players in the process. Trusts have been accused of aggressively defending their turf and of driving the policy agenda in the absence of firm leadership and vision from purchasing authorities. There is indeed often little connection between purchasers' strategies and those of their principal providers who continue to peddle cherished schemes regardless of whether purchasers wish to support them. Working together, though not too cosily, seems the only tenable option in the longer term. One such attempt is the West Yorkshire Initiative set up in 1993 to facilitate the strategic shift to primary and community care across purchasers and providers in the West Yorkshire area (see Box 2.7 for details, and Hunter 1993c).

Whatever the potential of the NHS reforms, in particular their focus on health gain, they run the danger 'of being lost in a thicket of rules, contradictory directives, confusing information, and neutralizing vested interests' (Light 1994, p. 9). Arguably, the original emphasis on competition between providers, particularly trusts, has frustrated efforts to purchase or commission services

Box 2.7
The West Yorkshire initiative

> The Initiative which ran from May 1993 to October 1994 was supported by Yorkshire (then Northern and Yorkshire) RHA and the NHS Executive. It was managed by the four purchaser authorities in West Yorkshire. It was located in an independent academic centre, the Nuffield Institute for Health, University of Leeds. The Initiative's purpose was twofold:
>
> ◆ To seek to forecast the likely health issues of the 21st century and provide a resource to those seeking this information
> ◆ To assist the four health authorities which make up West Yorkshire (covering a population of 2.1 million) to find ways of working together to tackle the major health care problems they face and which cannot be resolved by any single authority acting in isolation.
>
> The Initiative was *not*
>
> ◆ a supra-district layer of bureaucracy
> ◆ going to produce a blueprint or final report.
>
> The Initiative team operated as facilitators, enablers and brokers seeking opportunities to develop a shared vision of what purchasing *across* West Yorkshire means.
> The Initiative has completed or launched the following:
>
> ◆ a geographical mapping exercise of service use in West Yorkshire
> ◆ supporting experiments in developing the new agenda in primary care
> ◆ service reviews in renal, neonatal, cancer and cardio-thoracic services
> ◆ keeping close to Community Health Councils.

for health. Few would disagree that the aims of the reforms can only be realized through strong purchasing. Otherwise providers will capture the newly created markets and use monopolistic powers to drive up costs and frustrate the reforms. It is possible that this has already happened in many parts of the country thus making the purchasers' task more difficult. On the other hand, there is little evidence available to demonstrate that a shift from secondary to primary care will necessarily lead to health gains. In the absence of such evidence, the strategy can be little more than an act of faith. It fuels concern, even if it has no basis in policy, that the aim of the shift is not to improve the quality of care but to save money.

Purchasing may be top of the government's agenda for the time being but if it fails to deliver within a reasonable time span conceivably its place on the agenda will be taken by some other policy initiative. The problem lies in knowing what delivering means in this context as there is no coherent strategic framework at the centre to serve as a benchmark. Indeed, the DoH and NHSE each have their own ideas about strategy which has given rise to tensions, if not conflicts, between different policies. For example, elements of the performance management framework, such as the **efficiency index** (with its emphasis on secondary care through-put), conflict with the shift of emphasis envisaged in *Health of the Nation* from hospital treatment to primary care prevention of illness and health promotion (Kerr *et al.* 1993). A further conflict is evident in the reforms' emphasis on improving services and choice for individuals. This may not fit well with the population-based commissioning role of DHAs. Too great a focus on the needs of the individual inevitably leads to inequity.

Central policies and priorities are important in setting a context in which the market is to be managed and regulated. A corporate strategic framework has therefore been proposed to ensure that strategic policies at the centre are not pursued in isolation but are linked coherently (Kerr *et al.* 1993). A possible NHS strategic framework is given in Figure 2.3 and described in Box 2.8.

SUMMARY

The central dilemma for the government is the sheer unpredict-ability of the forces it has unleashed. In 1991, the NHS and community care services were launched on a huge experiment and no-one knows what the likely outcome will be for the creation of health strategy. Light quotes a senior manager as saying that the government 'threw cards into the air' (Light 1993, p. 9). Whether these forces can be managed and steered in a coherent direction through a strategic framework, which is presently piecemeal, is a major issue for ministers and the NHS Chief Executive.

At the end of the day, the question is whether an internal market will prove more or less successful in bringing about improvements in health care provision and in the status of

Box 2.8
Functional strategies
for the NHS: key
themes

Functional area	Key themes

Environmental context	◆ Developments in other sectors that may have an impact on the planning and delivery of health care; e.g.:
	  – European policy
	  – legal issues
	  – environmental legislation and guidelines
	  – local government changes
	  – economic outlook

Finance	◆ Resource allocation policies ◆ Arrangements for capital allocation and capital charging ◆ Cash flow management ◆ Standards and protocols for financial probity and audit ◆ Outline structure for costing and pricing systems
Organization	◆ Type of market ◆ The role of market management and regulation ◆ The future of GP fundholding ◆ Roles and freedoms of different organizations in the NHS ◆ Organization development for commissioning, NHS trusts and GP fundholders
Human resources	◆ Long-term view of the work force, its skills, knowledge and experience base ◆ Medical staffing policy and procedures ◆ Opportunity 2000 ◆ Conditions of work and broad pay and reward practices ◆ Education, training and development, including the future of Working Paper 10 monies ◆ Performance management processes (micro-level)
Cultural issues and communications	◆ The relationship between clinicians and managers ◆ Communication of the NHS objectives and values and how they should inform decision making ◆ Equal opportunities/encouraging cultural diversity ◆ Empowering patients ◆ Partnerships between purchasers–providers and other agencies
Information	◆ Opportunities offered by changing technology; e.g. smart cards and bar codes, networks, etc. ◆ Workload classification ◆ Quality assurance in information ◆ Developing capabilities across the range of data gathering and information handling (including analysis, presentation and use) ◆ Review of reporting arrangements

Source: Adapted from Kerr *et al.* (1993)

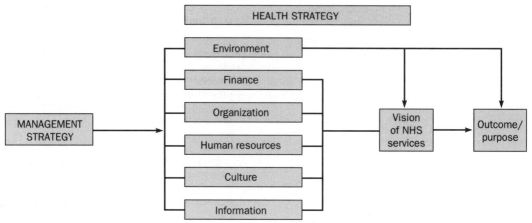

Figure 2.3
A strategic framework for the NHS
(*Source*: Kerr *et al.* 1993)

*Dr's Autonomy
Needs
Challenging*

people's health, or whether central planning and direction remain necessary to achieve these ends.

The problem, in the past as now, may not have been the structures and systems but the absence of will to challenge entrenched interests, notably the medical profession, and effect real change. That remains the central political and strategic issue, and neither a top-down, command and control system of strategic management nor a decentralized, managed market can in themselves resolve it. To succeed, it requires sustained political and managerial leadership.

**FURTHER
READING**

◆ Pettigrew, A., Ferlie, E. and McKee, L. (1992), *Shaping Strategic Change*, Sage, London.

◆ Rathwell, R. (1987), *Strategic Planning in the Health Sector*, Croom Helm, London.

◆ Robinson, R. and Le Grand, J. (Eds) (1994), *Evaluating the NHS Reforms*, King's Fund, London.

◆ Tilley, I. (Ed.) (1993), *Managing the Internal Market*, Paul Chapman, London.

REFERENCES

Allison, G.T. (1971), *Essence of Decision*. Boston: Little Brown.

Audit Commission (1993), *Taking Care: Progress with Care in the Community*, Health and Personal Social Services Bulletin no. 1. London: HMSO.

Baeza, J., Salt, D. and Tilley, I. (1993), Four providers' strategic responses and the internal market. In: Tilley, I. (Ed.), *Managing the Internal Market*. London: Paul Chapman.

Barnard, K. (1977), Promises, patients and politics: the conflicts of the NHS. In: Barnard, K. and Lee, K. (Eds), *Conflicts in the National Health Service.* London: Croom Helm.

Barnard, K. (1991), Trends in health care: beyond market economics. A reflection on 40 years past and 10 years future. In: Bengoa, R. and Hunter D. J. (Eds), *New Directions in Managing Health Care.* Leeds: World Health Organization and Nuffield Institute for Health Services Studies.

Cm 555 (1989), *Working for Patients.* London, HMSO.

Cm 849 (1989), *Caring for People.* London, HMSO.

Cm 1986 (1992), *The Health of the Nation: A Strategy for Health in England.* London, HMSO.

Cmnd 7615 (1979), *Report of Royal Commission on the NHS.* London, HMSO.

Department of Health (1991), *Research for Health: A Research and Development Strategy for the NHS.* London: HMSO.

Department of Health (1993a), *Managing the New NHS.* A background document. London: DoH.

Department of Health (1993b), *Research for Health.* London: DoH.

Department of Health (1993c), *Community Care.* EL(93)119. London: DoH.

Department of Health and Social Services (1976), *Priorities for Health and Personal Social Services in England.* London: HMSO.

Edwards, B. (1993), *The National Health Service: A Manager's Tale 1946-1992.* London: Nuffield Provincial Hospitals Trust.

Enthoven, A.C. (1985), *Reflections on the Management of the NHS: An American Looks at Incentives to Efficiency in Health Services Management in the UK.* London: Nuffield Provincial Hospitals Trust.

Evans, T. (1987a), Strategic response to environmental turbulence. In: Stocking, B. (Ed.), *In Dreams Begin Responsibility.* London: King's Fund.

Evans, T. (1987b), Managing service changes with declining resources. In: Stocking, B. (Ed.), *In Dreams Begin Responsibility.* London: King's Fund.

Glennerster, H., Matsaganis, M. and Owens, P. with Hancock, S. (1994), *Implementing GP Fundholding.* Buckingham: Open University Press.

Griffiths, R. (1983), *Report: NHS Management Inquiry.* London: DHSS.

Harrison, S., Hunter, D.J., Johnston, I. and Wistow, G. (1989), *Competing for Health: A Commentary on the NHS Review,* Nuffield Institute Report no. 1. Leeds: Nuffield Institute for Health Services Studies.

Harrison, S., Hunter, D.J. and Nicholson, N. *et al.* (1991), *Health Before Health Care.* London: Institute for Public Policy Research.

Health Service Commissioner (1994), *Second Report for Session 1993-94: Failure to Provide Long Term NHS Care for a Brain-Damaged Patient.* London: HMSO.

Health Services Management Unit (1992), *Caring for the Community in the 21st Century: Integrated Purchasing of Public Services.* Macclesfield: Greenhalgh & Co.

Hood, C.A. (1991), Public management for all seasons? *Public Administration,* 69:3.

Hunter, D.J. (1993a), Protect and survive, *Health Service Journal,* 103:21.

Hunter, D.J. (1993b), *Rationing Dilemmas in Healthcare,* Research Paper no. 8. Birmingham: National Association of Health Authorities and Trusts.

Hunter, D.J. (1993c), Purchasing for health in the 21st century, *NHS Trust Conference Bulletin*. Leeds: Simpson Curtis.

Johnson, G. (1987), *Strategic Change and the Management Process*. Oxford: Basil Blackwell.

Kerr, R., Liddell, A. and Spry, C. (1993), *Towards an Effective NHS*. London: Office for Public Management.

Le Grand, J. and Bartlett, W. (1993), *Quasi-Markets in Social Policy*. Basingstoke: Macmillan.

Light, D.W. (1994), *Strategic Challenges in Joint Commissioning: Challenges and Strategic Issues in Comparative Perspective*. London: North West Thames RHA.

McKevitt, D. (1992), Strategic management in public services. In: Willcocks, L. and Harrow, J. (Eds), *Rediscovering Public Services Management*. Maidenhead: McGraw-Hill.

Mawhinney, B. and Nichol, D. (1993), *Purchasing for Health: A Framework for Action*. Leeds: NHS Management Executive.

Maynard, A. (1993), Creating competition in the NHS: Is it possible? Will it work? In: Tilley, I. (Ed.), *Managing the Internal Market*. London: Paul Chapman.

Miller, R.H. and Luft, H.S. (1991), Perspective, diversity and transition in health insurance plans, *Health Affairs*, 37.

Mintzberg, H. (1988), Opening up the definition of strategy. In: Quinn, J. B. *et al*. (Eds), *The Strategy Process: Concepts, Contexts and Cases*. New Jersey: Prentice Hall.

Mintzberg, H. (1990), *Mintzberg on Management*. London: Free Press.

Newchurch (1992), *Acute Hospitals – A Case for Treatment*. London.

NHS Executive (1994), *Developing NHS Purchasing and GP Fundholding*. EL(94)79. Leeds: NHSE.

Parston, G. (Ed.) (1986), *Managers as Strategists*. London: King's Fund.

Pettigrew, A., Ferlie, E. and McKee, L. (1992), *Shaping Strategic Change*. London: Sage.

Pietroni, R. (1993), General practitioners and the market. In: Tilley, I. (Ed.), *Managing the Internal Market*. London: Paul Chapman.

Rathwell, T. (1987), *Strategic Planning in the Health Sector*. London: Croom Helm.

Richardson, A., Duggan, M. and Hunter, D.J. (1994), *Adapting to New Tasks: The Role of Public Health Physicians in Purchasing Health Care*. Leeds: Nuffield Institute for Health.

Robinson, J. and Wistow, G. (1993), *All Change, No Change? Community Care Six Months On*. London: Nuffield Institute for Health and King's Fund Centre.

Robinson, R. and Le Grand, J. (Eds) (1994), *Evaluating the NHS Reforms*. London: King's Fund.

Schon, D. (1973), *Beyond the Stable State*. Harmondsworth: Penguin.

Smith, S.R. and Lipsky, M. (1992), Privatisation in health and human services: a critique, *Journal of Health Politics, Policy and Law*, 17:233.

Social Services Committee (1989), *Resourcing the NHS: the Government's Plans for the Future of the NHS*. Eighth Report, Session 1988–89, HC214-III. London: HMSO.

Tilley, I. (Ed.) (1993), *Managing the Internal Market*. London: Paul Chapman.

Trent RHA (1992), *Private Sector Lessons for the NHS*. Sheffield, Trent RHA.

Welsh Health Planning Forum (1989a), *Strategic Intent and Direction for the NHS in Wales*. Cardiff: Welsh Office NHS Directorate.

Welsh Planning Forum (1989b), *Local Strategies for Health: A New Approach to Strategic Planning*. Cardiff: Welsh Office NHS Directorate.

Wistow, G., Knapp, M., Hardy, B. *et al*. (1992), From providing to enabling: local authorities and the mixed economy of social care, *Public Administration*, 70:25.

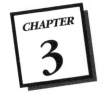

FINANCIAL MANAGEMENT REFORM IN THE NHS

CHAPTER 3

John J. Glynn

OBJECTIVES

- ◆ To show how financial management in the NHS has developed to meet the needs of the internal market.

- ◆ To describe the pattern of financial information available in the NHS, and how this has been changed to be more useful for service management.

- ◆ To introduce financial techniques which can be used to support decision-making.

- ◆ To describe the key processes of costing, pricing, budgeting and controlling services.

INTRODUCTION

As might be expected following the radical reforms of recent years in the NHS, particularly the shift from administration to management of the service and the introduction of the **internal market**, the financial management of the NHS has had to change fairly radically in order to meet the new requirements. Such reforms of financial practice and processes were long overdue and were really needed regardless of the change in management philosophy arising out of the Griffiths inspired reforms of the 1980s. This basic shift had been to move away from the emphasis on rather 'global' and hierarchical cost control as the primary means of financial management towards a broader approach whereby greater attention is paid to locally determined management accounting systems that are more responsive to local management needs.

As we all know, the NHS was established in 1948 with a mandate that promised unlimited, free medical care of the best possible standard for the entire population. However this promise lasted barely twelve months. Costs soared out of control in Nye Bevan's first year as Minister of Health – so much so that Stafford Cripps, the then Chancellor, announced in his 1948 budget that the Treasury would set a ceiling on NHS expenditure and that, henceforth, the British public would be entitled to as much free care as could be afforded within this economic limit. So when commentators decry the current lack of resourcing in the NHS we need to reflect that we have in fact had an undersupply of medical care, and hence rationing, for the best part of fifty years.

For clinicians it is important to appreciate the background against which current financial management reforms are taking place. This is necessary in order to appreciate both the financial information requirements needed in the NHS of the 1990s and the major change in the nature of the accountabilities whereby clinicians are expected to take a much more proactive and informed part in the decision-making process. The financial management of the NHS has moved from a position where operational costs were allocated downwards and successful performance was perceived as staying within the target allocation. **Capital funding** for intrastructural investment was managed at a regional level such that capital was perceived by provider units as a 'free' good.

When, as part of the overall financial strategy for the public sector, the government introduced cash limits and cash planning as a means of limiting waste and improving efficiency, there was little concerted effort to improve the quality of financial information for localized decision making. With the introduction of the NHS internal market this has had to change. Now financial accountability, in the broad sense, has been devolved down to purchaser and provider units. Hospital trusts and GP **fundholders** are responsible for both revenue and capital expenditure. Trusts have also been granted **external financing limits** (EFLs); that is, the ability to borrow from outside the NHS a certain level of funds for additional capital expenditure. Figure 3.1 is not a conventional organizational chart but rather an attempt to illustrate the major NHS funding flows as from 1992-93. Whilst accountability is being devolved down to the new managers of the internal market, it is important to note that the public sector health market is still subject to an overall cash limit and hospitals are subject to stringent central regulations with respect to the important questions of pricing, capital investment and the range of services to be offered.

This chapter first reviews the background against which current financial management reforms are taking place. Then, in turn, it looks at what new costing techniques are being introduced, the pricing of health care, the development of behaviourally sound budgetary planning and control systems, capital appraisal, capital maintenance, performance indicators, financial reporting and audit. It concludes with a short review of the influence of contract management on financial management.

Figure 3.1
Proposed major NHS
funding flows,
1992–93

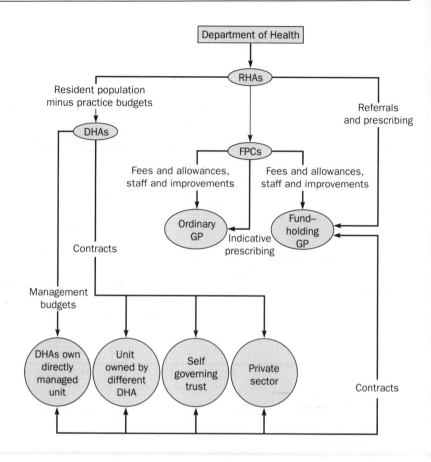

TRADITIONAL
FINANCIAL
INFORMATION

Throughout the early decades of the NHS the main emphasis, as far as financial management was concerned, was on hierarchical cost control. From 1948 to 1974 the (then) Ministry of Health required every hospital authority in England and Wales to report by the end of each month on the previous month's expenditure on all the main 'subjective' (or input) cost headings, and the cumulative expenditure from 1 April, compared with an appropriate proportion of the approved annual budget. Half-way through the year, revised estimates were called for which could be adjusted to take account of over- or underspendings which could not be avoided. For 26 years these forms were used, subject to minor modifications. The subjective analysis of expenditure had the merit of being simple to update as, for example, all cleaners' wages were collectively grouped under the heading 'domestic salaries and wages'. No attempt was made to classify costs to departments, clinics, wards, etc. so that there was no clear 'picture' of the pattern of expenditure incurred by a diverse range of activities. With the health reorganization of 1973, **'functional'** (or **cost centre**) accounting was introduced. Even allowing for this change two major omissions still occurred:

♦ Capital expenditure was treated as though it were a 'free good' as it was not formerly recorded as a part of operational expenditure.

♦ It was not possible to consider aspects of patient costing to recognize more discreetly how certain treatments and processes cost significantly more than other approaches.

Annual returns continued to be made to the Department of Health, and hospitals, unlike other public sector bodies, did not produce a summary financial report for public discussion and debate.

From the early 1970s greater attention was given to improving overall financial management within the NHS. To date the expansion of health care provision had been largely haphazard and unplanned and there was no overall policy for equalizing the scale and accessibility of health care resources across the country. The Resource Allocation Working Party (RAWP) was established with an objective to 'provide equal access to care'. Reporting in 1976, the RAWP proposed that funds should henceforth be allocated to regions according to a formula designed to establish an equitable criteria of need. RAWP targets were set for both revenue and capital expenditure. Those readers wishing for a more detailed overview of how this system was supposed to work should refer to references DHSS (1976) and DHSS (1980).

The 1980s saw an increasing interest in 'specialty costing'. For example the Körner Committee (DHSS, 1984) sought, through Working Party F, to improve and make more meaningful cost information. This working party provided five criticisms of the (then) existing financial information systems (Box 3.1).

Various approaches to costing were considered: patient costing; diagnostic group costing; clinical team costing; and specialty costing. Körner opted for specialty costing, and in particular the

Box 3.1
Five criticisms identified by the Körner Committee

♦ Financial information did not provide the cost of treating different groups of patients (i.e. translating the 'input' of resources into the 'outputs' of health care).

♦ Costs produced in the uniform departmental (functional) analysis did not reflect local budgetary responsibilities.

♦ Hospital classifications, under the costing system, did not account for the substantial variations in case-mix which existed between hospitals of the same type.

♦ Financial information was often of suspect validity, particularly when apportionment was required to produce patient analysis.

♦ Financial information was tardy – particularly for budget holders who require information to control expenditure.

'sampling' approach based on the work of Professor Charles Magee of Cardiff University. For a more detailed discussion of the history and development of specialty costing see Hillman (1984), Perrin (1988) and Glynn (1993).

For three decades attention has been paid to costing and, to a lesser extent, budgeting as a means of controlling health care expenditure. Management and professional accountability, in economic terms, was far from clear. Whatever accounting reforms might have taken place, the NHS still operated by **consensus management** which critics believed led to weakly determined decisions within health authorities. There were often voids between the administration and the clinical and other professional support disciplines.

The NHS Management Inquiry (DHSS, 1983), the **Griffiths Report**, was very critical of this consensus management approach, and recommended it be replaced by **activity-based management**. Central to the reforms initiated by Griffiths was the notion of the 'general manager' working alongside clinicians who would henceforth become involved in the management process and budgeting. Other issues which would also involve the general manager and clinicians included attention to quality improvement and consumer participation and the introduction of better personnel management – including appraisal, manpower planning and the operation of incentive schemes. The Griffiths recommendations formed the foundation for 'Working for Patients' (Cm 555) published as a White Paper in 1989.

All general managers are appointed on short-term rolling contracts, the renewal of which is dependent upon annual appraisals of their performance. General managers may also receive performance related pay. Other health authority staff are responsible to general managers, although the status of consultants, as set out in Cm 555, is slightly ambiguous. Traditionally most consultants were employed by regional rather than district health authorities but with the disbandment of regions and the creation of hospital trusts it is clear that consultants are now much more closely aligned to the performance of the trust within which they reside.

This policy review was a fundamental shakeup of the health care management process, not the least of which was the new funding systems introduced as a result of the creation of the internal market and the purchaser–provider based model of health care provision. Fundamentally, the majority of funding now resides with locally based purchasers of whom the GP fundholders are the dominant group – a model that creates a system of internal markets in which the NHS care institutions compete with each other in order to produce a more efficient and responsive service to users.

All significant hospitals are now self-governing trusts, free of district control, employing their own staff, including consultant

Private Financing Ltd

medical staff, and able to raise capital in the private sector subject to an external financial limit (EFL) set by the National Health Service Executive. Some readers will say that these reforms are the result of political conviction. Others will say that there is an intellectual basis to Cm 555 and that this document contains much of the ideas of Enthoven (1985).

Enthoven considered that the separation of the purchasing and providing roles in health care would mean that purchasers 'could buy services from producers who offered good value' and that the 'bargaining leverage' of being able to buy outside would produce better performance from the internal providers. Unlike the rigorous detail given to costing processes in the previous three decades, the thrust of Cm 555 was devoid of detailed prescription. An approach was outlined, certain principles were enunciated and both purchasers and providers are now broadly free to develop their own 'tailored' financial management systems. Box 3.2 shows basic rules against which systems are to be developed.

Box 3.2
Basic rules for financial management systems

- The price of patient treatment is to be considered as the full cost – that is, including an allowance for associated capital costs, such as buildings and equipment, which are no longer to be treated as a 'free good'.

- Purchasers and providers have to achieve balanced budgets year on year.

- All levels of management must demonstrate that funds are prudently allocated, expenditure strictly controlled and performance critically examined.

Understanding Contracting important

On the one hand these are issues that are very much part of the contracting process. On the other hand, service delivery must be demonstrated – hence the requirement for a new thinking in the financial management process, one that clearly links to the quality and timeliness of service delivery.

As far as general managers and clinicians are concerned there is a critical need to understand new costing techniques, to be able to develop and operate behaviourally sound budgetary planning and control systems, and to understand the influence of contracting on the both of these.

MAKING FINANCIAL INFORMATION MORE USEFUL

We have already looked at the notion of subjective (or input) costs and functional costs whereby these subjective costs are allocated to particular wards, departments, activities etc. It is, though, important to distinguish other ways of analysing costs. Four other useful approaches to cost classification are:

◆ by service;
◆ by behaviour;
◆ by controllability;
◆ by relevance.

Each of these approaches is briefly discussed in turn.

Costs by service   **Classification of costs by service** simply answers the question: What are our particular services costing us? There are two elements to such a calculation:

◆ the direct costs of providing care, such as staff costs, drugs etc.;
◆ the indirect costs or **overheads** not directly attributable to one particular service but needing to be apportioned in such a way as to ensure that they are charged to the client.

The overhead costs must include a charge for the capital assets also used. The NHS Executive does provide some guidance on overhead cost allocation, but a number of interpretations are possible and this can lead to competing hospitals producing markedly different prices for treatment which each would be more than prepared to justify. When it comes to the process of allocating overheads there is no 'right way', only pragmatic solutions. The only other guidance provided by the department is that contract prices should take account of all costs, including depreciation at current cost and 6% interest on capital assets, and that there should be no cross-subsidization of services and treatments.

It was the inability of many providers to detail their costs in the approved fashion that led to the initial large volume of 'block contracts' which clearly often had the provider at a disadvantage.

Costs by behaviour   **Classification of costs by behaviour** allows managers and clinicians to address the question: How will our total costs change as a result of an increase or decrease in the level of our activities? Typically, costs can be divided into three types:

◆ **fixed**, unchanging regardless of the level of activity;
◆ **semi-fixed** (or step costs) which are fixed for a given range of activity;
◆ **variable**, changing directly as activity increases or decreases.

For most general purposes we can assume that variable costs are linear. This is not exactly right but is sufficiently true so as to make our discussion fairly uncomplicated. Fixed costs will include many overhead costs, including the cost of capital, light and heat etc.; but can also include some staff costs. Other salary costs, for example nursing costs, may be semi-fixed. Often many costs are fixed as a result of management action. For example, some direct staffing costs could be changed to sessional, and thus variable, cost.

This basic distinction into fixed and variable costs is also termed '**marginal costing**'. It is a simple yet powerful tool since it enables managers and clinicians to determine easily the level of activity necessary to cover all costs.

To illustrate this concept we can look at a simple formula. Suppose that TS stands for *total sales income*, TVC for *total variable cost* and TFC for *total fixed cost*. We can think in terms of 'sales income' because contracts are such that providers sell services to purchasers. The *surplus* S (or *deficit* D) is then given by the formula:

$$S \text{ (or D)} = TS - TVC - TFC. \qquad (1)$$

The break-even point occurs when sales income covers all direct and indirect costs, when S is zero. At this point we can rearrange the formula as follows:

$$TS - TVC = TFC \qquad (2)$$

To determine the number of units that have to be sold to break even (e.g. the number of patients treated), we can develop a third formula. If the *unit selling price* is US and the *unit variable cost* is UVC, then:

$$\text{Number of units to break even} = \frac{TFC}{US - UVC}. \qquad (3)$$

Accountants and economists use the term '**contribution**' to describe the difference between the unit selling price and the unit variable cost.

When you understand the principles of **marginal costing** then you can also appreciate why, fairly quickly, many block contracts moved to being within defined upper and lower limits of activity. This approach is much more equitable to both purchaser and provider. Referring to the example in Box 3.3, if a purchaser had contracted for 50 patients to attend this clinic and only 30 were actually sent, there might be some grievance at having to pay the total cost of £10 000 (£200 × 50). However, from the point of view of the provider, resources had to be made available for this contractor and whilst 20 patients did not turn up some fixed costs were incurred. It would be equitable to charge the purchaser £8400, a saving of £1600 (£80 variable costs × 20). Conversely, if the purchaser, having during the course of the year become aware that the provider has some spare capacity, actually wanted to buy additional clinic sessions it would be somewhat unfair to have to pay the previous price of £200 since at this rate all fixed costs are being recovered. The variable cost rate of £80 would be more equitable.

Box 3.3
A simple example

> A particular clinic's unit treatment price per patient is £200, based on a unit variable cost of £80 and a monthly fixed cost of £12 000. Using formula (3) we can see that it is necessary to treat 100 patients a month in order to cover all the clinic's costs. If, for example, the clinic's consultant wishes to upgrade the technical facilities in the clinic such that monthly fixed costs would rise to £15 000 per month, it would be necessary to treat 125 patients per month in order to cover all costs. Could this be done? In the common parlance, can an additional number of patients be provided in the market?
>
> In part this question is answered by whether or not the purchasers agree to fund additional patients to this clinic and whether or not rival providers can provide an equal service for a lower price. Given the competitive environment that most providers find themselves in, it is vital that unit contribution is either maximized in order to reduce the risk of covering fixed costs, or that fixed costs are reduced commensurate with a reduction in unit contribution.

In fact this example is rather simplistic to illustrate the mechanics of the costing technique. Contracting rules state 'cost = price' over the anticipated annual demand for a particular service and that limited marginal work can be undertaken if spare capacity arises. Contract prices have to be announced at the beginning of the financial year and are not usually subject to revision.

Costs by controllability

With respect to the **classification of costs by controllability** the question to be determined is: Who is responsible (and thus accountable) for the costs that are being incurred? The issue here is that all too often budget holders receive budget statements which contain costs that they cannot control or influence. Are managers motivated by having statements that contain many apportioned and reallocated charges for which they cannot account directly, when the bottom line is that they are expected to have a balanced budget at the end of the year? The author is convinced that budgets used for the purposes of management control should only contain

Box 3.4
Example

> Bought-in services are usually at a known standard price. It might be that a clinician requires a certain radiological test for a patient. This might require two X-rays of a certain type. The cost charged to the clinician is a known standard charge and if, for example, a radiologist had unexpectedly to do three X-rays then the inefficiency would not be recharged to the clinician.

expenditure lines that the manager can influence. Controllability varies with the hierarchical structure of the institution, the seniority of the manager and the basic management processes by which services are provided. Things have improved in recent years.

There will be more to say on the nature of controllable costs when we come to consider the notion of 'flexible' budgeting.

Costs by relevance   The final cost classification to be considered in this section is that of **cost by relevance**. This is a vital concept when considering the future deployment of limited resources. The question therefore to be determined is: What would the cost consequences of pursuing a particular course of action be in the future? For future decision making we need, when considering alternative strategies, to consider only differential costs and to recognize the notion of '**opportunity cost**'. Opportunity cost can be defined as the cost of the best alternative foregone.

Box 3.5
Example

> A clinician may be paid £15 per hour irrespective of whether he or she sees patient A or B, and yet the price attached to patient B may be considerably higher. If the overall charge for treating patient A produces a contribution of £80 and for patient B £240, and given that the clinician would have spent a total of two hours with patient A and three hours with patient B, the opportunity cost (per hour) of the clinician is £40 per hour with patient A and £80 per hour with patient B. What the clinician actually receives per hour is irrelevant from working out his or her economic utility.

This costing technique is vital when deciding on the mix of services being provided by a provider with finite and scarce resources. Clearly it makes sense to optimize as far as possible the utility of scarce resources and accept the fact that, to put it bluntly, some patient treatments may not be economic.

Clearly the notion of 'opportunity cost' will sit uncomfortably with some clinicians since they will not want to discriminate between different classes of patients. More strategically, it is certainly true that some trusts are giving serious consideration to their skill mix and to the particular type of patient services they will offer in the future. Again, if there is a particular service that can be exploited it makes sense, from the trust's perspective, to do so.

For further discussion of basic costing techniques see Glynn, Perrin and Murphy (1994).

THE PRICING OF   The NHS Executive (**NHSE**) set out its approach on the pricing
HEALTH CARE   of contracts in October 1990. There were three fundamental principles:

◆ Contracts should generally be priced at cost.
◆ Contracts should take account of all costs including depreciation at current cost and 6% interest on capital assets.
◆ There should be no planned cross-subsidization.

Providers are given a wide degree of discretion in the detailed application of these principles but they are required to have documentation for audit purposes. Treatment price has to be announced in advance of the forthcoming financial year and to be based on anticipated activity for that year, including anticipated extra-contractual referrals and allowances for cost improvements over the year just ending. Marginal-cost contracts, of the type illustrated above, can only be written when unplanned spare capacity arises in excess of the assumed volume of service.

From the beginning, many providers had real problems arriving at the real full cost of services. There were particular difficulties with respect to the division of overheads. In addition, it soon became obvious that, for a variety of reasons, different providers were offering the same or similar treatment for vastly different prices. In the mind of the government, the market mechanism would resolve this issue since the inefficient providers would simply lose business. However, price differentials occurred for a number of reasons. Certainly some providers were inefficient, but other reasons arose because of different modes of service delivery and the basic accounting issues associated with the three principles outlined above. Could one hospital help it if its **capital infrastructure** was very different from a rival competitor's? Were all providers recovering costs in the same way? Often too many costs were indirect because their incidence was not properly traceable to particular treatments. The suspicion soon grew that astute providers wishing to sustain certain activities produced prices acceptable to the market and then arranged their cost allocations accordingly.

For the 1994/95 contracting round the NHSME felt that two areas of costing needed to be developed in order to improve the understanding of cost behaviour and thereby narrow the pricing differences that occurred as a result of providers adopting different accounting practices. It was their view that, in terms of **absorption costing**, a consistent approach to costing for contracting and the precision of cost analysis would be enhanced if:

◆ a minimum standard for each cost was identified as to its type – that is, direct, indirect and overhead;
◆ a more standardized approach to methods of apportionment for indirect costs and overheads was adopted;
◆ the proportion of costs directly charged to a product was increased.

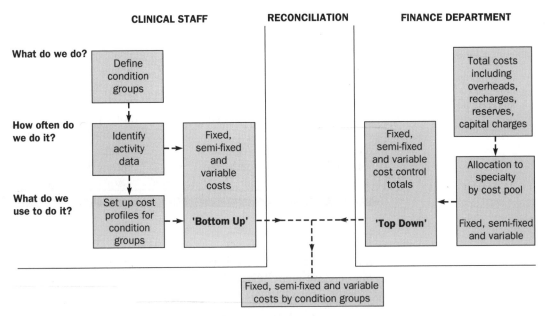

Figure 3.2
A pictorial summary of 'Top Down, Bottom Up, Reconciliation'

It was also suggested that the contracting process would be more flexible and responsive to changes in activity if the proportion of costs identified as fixed was reduced and the proportion of costs identified as variable was increased. Local budget costs must now conform to nationally recognized categories. A general approach has been recommended entitled 'Top Down, Bottom Up, Reconciliation'. Figure 3.2 is a pictorial summary of the methodology, the anticipated benefits of which are:

♦ ensuring that the more detailed data obtained in the Bottom Up analysis is used to refine the Top Down;
♦ assisting the annual business planning and budget-setting process;
♦ assisting in the development of more meaningful contract negotiations.

Guidance was also provided in order to ensure a consistent framework for contracting, thereby enabling both purchasers and providers to have a degree of confidence in the analysis of costs and cost behaviour changes in response to fluctuating activity levels. By way of illustration, the classifications given in Box 3.6 would probably be fairly well accepted by purchasers and providers alike. Such efforts by the NHSE should lead to less problems in determining treatment price.

Box 3.6
Standard cost
classifications

Description	Classification	Analysis
Consultant	Fixed	Direct
Senior Registrar	Semi-fixed	Direct
Biochemist	Semi-fixed	Indirect
Finance Director	Fixed	Overhead
Drugs/gases	Variable	Usually indirect, sometimes direct
Dressings	Variable	Direct
X-ray film	Variable	Usually indirect, sometimes direct

As stated earlier, capital is no longer treated as a 'free good'. A capital charge is included, generally as an overhead, in the cost of treatment. This charge is composed of two elements:

♦ *a charge for depreciation,* based on the current cost and not the historical cost of equipment used;
♦ *an interest charge,* determined by HM Treasury, currently 6%.

Naive clinicians often assume that the depreciation element of this charge provides them with a fund against which equipment can be replaced. Nothing could be further from the truth. Some of the funds generated are simply to support operational expenditure and capital funds are still available only on a competitive basis. The interest element represents a direct return required by government on its investment in the NHS. For donated assets there is no need to charge the interest element of the capital charge, but the NHSE regard it as prudent to depreciate such assets and take account of depreciation in their prices. If, for example, a donation was made for the benefit of a specific group of patients it would not be unreasonable for a lower price to be determined which would thereby allow expanded provision for other groups.

% imposed by Govt.

BUDGET PLANNING AND CONTROL

Budgetary control is a vital part of the financial management of any organization. Historically, as alluded to earlier, budgetary control has not been treated too seriously within the NHS. Line managers have not always agreed with the way the budget has been cast, what they can reasonably control and what they cannot, and senior management have only been concerned that the organization as a whole achieves a balanced budget. Many budget holders will be familiar with the nonsensical approach that penalizes those who underspend on their budget and rewards, in the next year, those who overspend by granting them an increase in budget.

Cannot Always Perceive Account for Extra Expenses

Often budget holders are not necessarily able to control the amount of activity that passes through their section. Reasons for this are diverse. Perhaps the person setting contracts has miscalculated anticipated volumes of activity. Perhaps, due to bad weather, there has been an unanticipated incidence of admissions of patients with respiratory problems. It would be a rare event if planned activity were to match actual activity. In most organizations, and the NHS is no exception, it is often the case that planning and operational activities are separate management functions. If this is so then it makes sense for trusts to provide a system of '**flexible budgeting**' as it is both equitable to individual managers and fair in determining areas to which senior management attention should be focused.

The more traditional approach fixes a budget in advance of the forthcoming financial year. This will be subdivided into 12 monthly units or 13 four-weekly reporting units. Let us, referring back to our earlier clinic example, suppose that a particular budget envisages that 100 patients will be seen each month by the clinic. In practice more or fewer patients will be seen each month. For example, if 110 patients have been seen it is obvious that the clinic's variable expenditure will be higher than budgeted for. Externally this appears bad yet the consultant knows that the team have actually treated 10% more patients that month.

With a system of flexible budgeting the monthly control report becomes a three-column report (see Figure 3.3). The overall, and frankly meaningless, variance is broken down into two separate classes of variance:

♦ **planning variances** for which managers with a planning responsibility should be held accountable;
♦ **operational variances** for which service providers should be held accountable

If our consultant treated 10% more patients then it is not unreasonable to suggest that the variable costs should have risen by 10%. The same would be true in reverse – if less than the target level of patients were seen then there should have been a commensurate saving in variable costs.

Figure 3.3
Variances in a flexible budget approach

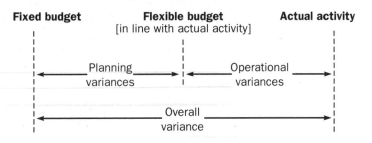

Fixed budget	Flexible budget [in line with actual activity]	Actual activity
Planning variances	Operational variances	
Overall variance		

Operational variances can be further subdivided into *price* (or rate) and *efficiency* variances. This subdivision is again useful as the consultant may not be responsible for establishing the pay levels of the team or for the purchase of various of the consumables such as drugs, CSSD packs etc. This sub-analysis is simply calculated as follows: (Actual unit cost × Actual units) less (Standard unit cost × Standard units for this level of activity) from which we derive:

♦ Price variance:
   (Actual unit cost − Standard unit cost) × Actual units
♦ Efficiency variance:
   (Actual units − Standard units) × Standard unit cost

Box 3.7
Example

> Let us suppose that part of the £80 of standard variable cost referred to earlier related to the need for a £5 CSSD pack for each patient treated, and that last month 105 patients were treated and the cost of CSSD packs was £556.20, representing actual usage of 108 packs at a charge of £5.15 each. The overall variance is:
>
> $$£556.20 - £525 = (£31.20).$$
>
> This overspend is not due entirely to the consultant's team. Firstly, the CSSD packs are costing more than was allowed for in the budget. The price variance is:
>
> $$(£5.15 - £5.00) \times 108 = (£16.20).$$
>
> However, for some reason three extra CSSD packs were used in the clinic, giving rise to an efficiency variance of:
>
> $$(108 - 105) \times £5.00 = (£15.00).$$
>
> The adverse price variance would be the concern of the supplies officer, whilst internal enquiries would need to be undertaken to see why three extra CSSD packs were used. This is a somewhat simple example but suffices to illustrate the process of variance analysis.

The introduction of a system of flexible budgeting is relatively inexpensive, being a simple spreadsheet application. However it does have the clear advantage of apportioning accountabilities to the lowest level possible and introduces the concept of explainable variances rather than overspends that cannot be truly attributed. Given the divorce of clinical responsibility from broader issues of contract management, a system of flexible budgeting is very much to the clinician's advantage. Clearly a move to this approach also means that those with slack budgets can no longer hide behind over-generous allocations of the past.

Flexible budgeting is simply a refinement of the more traditional approach to budgeting but it has the merit of being able to accommodate changes in activity month on month. It should also go without saying that such a system should only report on *controllable expenditure*.

Other budgetary systems have been promoted but have generally failed to achieve universal acceptance. Two such approaches were **programme budgeting** and **zero-base budgeting** (ZBB). Both systems failed because they tended to produce paper mountains and were too detailed. However, ZBB is sometimes used periodically rather than annually in recognition of the fact that traditional and flexible budgeting systems are incremental, year on year, and that periodically it is useful to pause and reflect on what is done, why, how it is done and for what cost. ZBB means that periodically we stop and recast particular budgets from scratch. This removes a level of complacency from the incremental nature of other budgetary systems. For further discussion on programme budgeting and ZBB see Glynn (1993).

CAPITAL APPRAISAL Over the years the NHS has not been terribly good at formally appraising, from an economic standpoint, where it should allocate its scarce capital funds. Funds were allocated to the former regional health authorities who often allocated them for a variety of reasons, but often as a result of lobbying. The preferred approach by both the Department of Health and Treasury was that such expenditure decisions should be formerly evaluated using a **discounted cashflow** technique called 'net present value' (NPV).

Given that costs and benefits occur over an extended period of the time, the NPV approach discounts future case flows by use of an imputed discount factor which should reflect the opportunity cost of capital. Future cash flows are then expressed in present value (today's) terms. The initial investment outlay is deducted from the sum of these present value cash flows to produce the NPV of a project; the decision rule is that all projects yielding a positive NPV should be accepted and all projects yielding a negative NPV should be rejected. The mechanics of the technique are not complicated, being akin to a compound interest calculation in reverse.

The opportunity cost discount rate is determined by the Treasury and is currently 6%, as used in determining the capital charge in the pricing of treatment. This rate is determined by Treasury actuaries and is based on the net-of-tax return achieved by low-risk medium-sized businesses in the private sector. Clearly as the economy improves and the profits earned in the private sector increase, so too will this rate since the opportunity principle adopted is that funds taken (taxed) from the private sector must be efficiently applied in the public sector.

Speculative

All elements of the NHS are being encouraged to ensure that all project appraisal is undertaken on the lines outlined above. In practice, we live in an uncertain environment where future events cannot be predicted with certainty and capital markets are far from perfect. As such the simplified approach outlined must be adapted to cope with these uncertainties but the discussion gets rather complicated and is outside the scope of the chapter. Specialist textbooks, such as Lumby (1994) and Collier, Cooke and Glynn (1987), provide further analysis of the problems that can arise and how to deal with them.

Capital maintenance

Capital asset management and maintenance is now devolved down to the provider level. In order for capital charges to be levied, capital asset registers have to be prepared and maintained. All directly managed hospitals are required to record and value all assets in excess of £1000. Only land is not subject to straight-line depreciation on current cost value. For many years the Treasury has accepted that valuing assets at their (original) historic cost does not really provide a measure of their actual value to the NHS. Each year therefore the assets recorded have to be *revalued* in terms of their current cost if being replaced and then depreciated in line with the period of time that the asset has been owned. Clearly problems arise as many assets are technologically obsolete before their physical life ends and proxy valuations may have to occur.

It is the responsibility of each trust to manage its own capital investment programme in line with its EFL. The EFL is determined on an individual basis and is based on the NHSE's view of how much capital can be serviced given the level of business and income generated by a particular trust.

PERFORMANCE INDICATORS

Despite the improvements taking place in the provision of financial information for management in the NHS, there is a need to supplement this information in order to demonstrate the full extent to which the providers of health care are also providing value for money (VFM). This oft quoted term can be thought of as comprising three elements (the three E's):

- Economy
- Efficiency
- Effectiveness.

Economy is relatively straightforward and is demonstrated by acquiring resources of an appropriate quality for the minimum cost. A sound system of flexible budgetary control, as outlined earlier, should ensure that due attention is paid to economy.

Efficiency means seeking to ensure that the maximum output is obtained from the resources devoted to a department or programme of treatment, or alternatively ensuring that only the minimum level of resources is devoted to a given level of output. An operation could be said to have increased in efficiency either if fewer inputs were used to produce a given amount of output, or a given level of input resulted in increased output.

Efficiency should not be confused with *productivity*. Efficiency is productivity relative to some standard, target or goal. Being efficient but not effective makes no sense, so efficiency measures in isolation have little benefit for the clinician. Efficiency measures clearly often impact directly on the effectiveness of health care. If, for example, the number of clinicians is reduced, implied efficiency (coping with more patients) is bound to have a detrimental effect on the quality of health care provided.

Effectiveness measures should be able to demonstrate that the output from any given activity is achieving the desired results. In health care such indicators should ideally be related to the outcome or impact of particular treatments – measures such as improved quality of life, re-admission etc.

Increasingly managers are being encouraged to develop performance indicators which they measure and monitor alongside their budgets. These pressures come from the NHSME, the purchasers and the Audit Commission, all of whom see performance indicators as an important part of the demonstration of management accountability. The golden rule for the development of such measures is that it is better to operate with a few key indicators that influence management behaviour rather than produce, *ex post*, a comprehensive list that never influence service delivery. The most problematic area is the development of effective performance measures. Most management information systems are not yet sufficiently sophisticated to generate the right data. Of course the effectiveness of treatment may not be determined for quite some time and therefore such measures will not directly impact on the clinician in a particular clinic or department. That is why medical audit and the use of protocols are useful surrogates for such performance indicators.

FINANCIAL REPORTING AND EXTERNAL AUDIT   As stated in the introduction, the units within the NHS have historically not produced annual financial reports of the type produced, for example, by local authorities. The usual reason for this was mainly that health care was entirely centrally funded. Whilst costs returns were provided for the Department of Health these were not public information. It is, however, true that local Finance Directors were generally very good at responding to *ad hoc* enquiries from the public and pressure groups etc.

With the introduction of the NHS internal market there is increasing pressure on purchasers and providers to produce annual accounting reports that are framed largely on the requirements of the Companies Acts in order to show a 'true and fair' view of, for example, a trust's or GP fundholder's financial affairs. The three key statements are a balance sheet, an income and expenditure statement (akin to the private sector profit and loss account) and a source and application of funds statement. Detailed guidance notes on the preparation of these statements are provided by the NHSE. As these reports become more commonplace in the 1990s additional information will be in the public arena for public debate.

SUMMARY: THE INFLUENCE OF CONTRACT MANAGEMENT ON FINANCIAL MANAGEMENT

There is little doubt that the introduction of the internal market – the contracting for health care – has led to a dramatic awareness of the need to improve financial management throughout the NHS. The most affected areas for this reform are undoubtedly the hospitals. Although the funds initially reside with the purchasers it is the providers who have had to reform their whole structure of financial management. We can already see clear evidence of this. As costing systems improve there are changes in the form of contracts being written. Block contracts are becoming cost-and-volume and cost-per-case contracts. The product definitions within contracts are becoming less focused on specialities and more based on procedures. Departmental budgets are starting in some instances to evolve into budgets based on product lines, flexed according to contracts with operational variances produced at the procedure level. Remembering issues of accountability discussed earlier, there is little benefit to allocating remote overheads to these budgets. Greater emphasis ought to be paid to the contributions that particular services and treatments make.

The challenge within the NHS is to develop accountants who readily understand the pressures of operating in the market and who appreciate that they are a support function to the providers of health care, in order to ensure that such providers are held more accountable for the services they offer and that value for money is achieved.

There are many who decry the shift to an NHS market; but it has to be remembered that, in a sense, good financial information ought to be neutral, and if the market were one day removed or restructured we ought not to remove the new financial reporting and control mechanisms.

It is also, and perhaps more contentiously, true that the medical profession can no longer divorce itself from the financial consequences of its actions. Perhaps one of the problems over the last five decades is that clinicians separated themselves to too great an extent from the management of the hospitals they worked in and they abdicated such responsibility to an administrative cadre who administered but who could not manage. Can one think of any other industry or profession where the key players sat on the sidelines when it came to management?

The purpose of this chapter is to create an awareness of the need for sound financial management throughout the NHS. Clinicians, increasingly involved in the management process, must demand relevant financial information and they must develop an understanding of how to work with such information. Accountants can provide financial information in many ways, clinicians must develop the skill of defining what information they need and for what purpose.

FURTHER READING

- ◆ Journals: Some of the issues are covered on a regular basis in the journals *Public Money and Management* and *Financial Accountability and Management*.

- ◆ Glynn, J., Perrin, J. and Murphy, M. (1994), *Accounting for Managers*, Chapman & Hall, London.

- ◆ NHS Management Executive (1993), *Costing for Contracting – The 1994–95 Round*, circular FDL(93) 59, London.

- ◆ Perrin, J. (1988), *Resource Management in the NHS*, VNR International/Chapman & Hall, London.

REFERENCES

Cm 555 (1989), *Working for Patients*. London: HMSO.

Collier, P.A., Cooke, T.E. and Glynn, J.J. (1988), *Financial and Treasury Management*. Oxford: Heinemann Professional.

Department of Health and Social Security (1976), *Sharing Resources of Health in England*. London: HMSO.

Department of Health and Social Security (1980), *Report of Advisory Group on Resource Allocation*. London: HMSO.

Department of Health and Social Security (1983), *Report of the NHS Management Inquiry* (Chairman: Sir Roy Griffiths). London: HMSO.

Department of Health and Social Security (1984), *Steering Group on Health Services Information – Report F* (Chairman: Edith Körner). London: HMSO.

Enthoven, A. (1985), *Reflections on the Management of the NHS*. London: Nuffield Hospitals Trust.

Glynn, J.J. (1993), *Public Sector Financial Control and Accounting*, 2nd edn. Oxford: Blackwell.

Glynn, J.J., Perrin, J. and Murphy, M.P. (1994), *Accounting for Managers*. London: Chapman & Hall.

Harrison, S., Hunter, D.J. and Pollitt, C. (1990), *The Dynamics of British Health Policy*. London: Unwin Hyman.

Hillman, R. (1984), *Speciality Costing in the National Health Service*. London: CIPFA.

Lumby, S. (1994), *Investment Appraisal and Financial Decisions*, 5th edn. London: Chapman & Hall.

NHS Management Executive (1993), *Costing for Contracting – The 1994/95 Round*, circular FDL(93)59, London.

Perrin, J. (1988), *Resource Management in the NHS.* London: VNR International/Chapman & Hall.

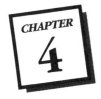

MANAGING PEOPLE AND TEAMS

CHAPTER 4

Alison Baker
and David A. Perkins

Alison Baker
and David A. Perkins

OBJECTIVES

- ◆ To describe the pattern of staffing in the NHS.

- ◆ To show how the context of the NHS constrains the options open to clinical managers in the management of staff.

- ◆ To show how the NHS internal market impacts on human resource management.

- ◆ To examine the contribution of staff management to service performance.

- ◆ To examine the importance for staff and services of effective management of change.

INTRODUCTION

While no-one would dispute that the quality of clinical care received by patients depends largely on the individuals and teams which provide that care, such issues do not form part of the medical curriculum. *Perhaps the hardest challenge to a clinical manager is the change from being a provider of care and advice to being a clinician and a manager of others.* The largest component of NHS expenditure is the salaries and wages of staff and one of the most hotly contested issues is the choice, training and organization of those people. It follows that one of the crucial challenges for the clinical manager is the effective management of people and teams.

This chapter provides the reader with a brief description of the pattern of staffing in the NHS and the rationale that underpins it. It attempts to show how discrete influences have changed this pattern both by design and by unintended impact. It describes how the basic arrangements for service planning and control influence the conditions under which staff work and determine the opportunities and constraints faced by clinical managers. It is possible to make a positive impact on the nature and quality of services by skilful staff management but such capabilities require careful nurturing and this chapter is intended to help in that process.

We will commence by looking at the NHS workforce and its composition, paying particular attention to changes in numbers, skills, and their balance. An examination of the key influences and constraints faced by managers will follow, pointing to their impact on the management of people. It sometimes appears that clinical managers are expected to achieve miracles 'with their hands tied behind their backs'. Thirdly, it is now the case that all NHS managers operate within the internal market which has direct impacts on managers at each level and from each profession. We will examine the market from the perspectives of government and the Management Executive who attempt to act as market managers, the purchasers, the service providers, and those in primary care who often act both as purchasers and providers. The next section will focus on the management of service performance or productivity. Performance often starts with conformance to contract but goes beyond simple issues of management control. Fifthly we will look at the management of people in change situations. Throughout, our concern is with the practising manager and particularly the clinician who has a management interest or responsibility.

THE NHS WORKFORCE

Describing the composition of the NHS workforce is no easy task. It is composed of full-time and part-time direct employees, external contractors, staff who work for more than one organization, and even some staff who work for two trusts which 'compete' within the internal market. Frequently staff have mixed loyalties to more than one organizational unit, undertake private practice or consultancy, and claim prime allegiance to patient, profession, or research and science rather than their employer. The categories in which staff are enumerated are complex and often owe as much to historical expedience as to rational analysis. Managers have often reacted to bureaucratic inflexibility, such as the **Whitley Council** process for determining staff pay and conditions, by adopting pragmatic rather than more rational solutions to staffing, job design, and how much staff are paid. Pragmatic actions have often solved immediate difficulties at the expense of creating differentials which later prove hard to justify or sustain. It is often difficult to identify consistent staffing patterns by institutional type, and this may be a result of the comparatively weak status and performance of the personnel function in the NHS as well as the wide range of hospitals and other institutions which have resulted from piecemeal growth. Indeed, painful experiences such as the nurse regrading exercise of the late 1980s reinforce the view that within the market, institutions and authorities should be free to develop a staffing pattern which maximizes productivity, reduces costs, but does not damage the national pool of skilled labour. It is likely that,

[margin note: Mixed Loyalties.]

[margin note: Fixing wages + cost of this]

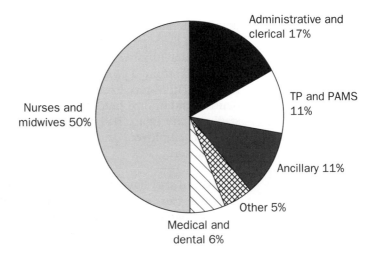

within the constraints of professional regulatory bodies, the market will increase the variety of staffing patterns.

In our interpretation of the patterns of NHS staffing we should be aware of changes in definitions, counting practices and the staff audits on which such figures are compiled. We should look to large trends rather than marginal variations, and there may be important questions for which the desired data are not available in a reliable form. Nonetheless some important conclusions can be drawn.

Figure 4.1 shows the broad proportions of staff working in the NHS in 1991, and Box 4.1 shows how these have changed since 1981. The figures are based on **whole-time equivalents** and are abstracted from *Social Trends* (1993). This period included a significant reorganization of management structures in 1982 and a more important change in management processes and institutional structures following the introduction of general management from 1985 onwards. The White Paper (Cm 555, 1989) and associated

Box 4.1
The pattern of staffing
in the NHS in the
United Kingdom, 1981
and 1991

*Staff
Pattern.*

	1981	1991
	(thousands)	
Medical and dental staff	49.7	57.8
Nursing and midwifery	492.8	501.3
Professional and technical (including PAMS)	80.2	106.5
Administrative and clerical	133.3	172.7
Ancillary staff	220.1	115.1
Other non-medical staff	56.2	53.2
TOTALS	1032.2	1006.6

developments at the end of the decade heralded the creation of trusts and the separation of purchasers and providers.

The total number of staff employed in the NHS had fallen marginally from 1 032 200 in 1981 to 1 006 600 in 1991 (UK figures). This figure excludes contractors for services such as GPs, dentists and optical practitioners. In 1981 there were 54 300 such staff and the figure had risen to 61 100 in 1991. The distinction between employees and contractors has important management implications:

- ◆ Salaried staff have broad job descriptions, terms and conditions which can be altered using set procedures, allowing management significant freedom of action.
- ◆ Contractors operate to an agreement negotiated collectively with their representatives which may include agreed variations to meet local circumstances. Changing the services offered by contractors takes place by renegotiating the contract or by offering fee-for-service payments to secure various services. More detailed discussion of this issue can be found in Chapter 7.

Nurses and midwives   The largest component of the directly employed workforce by some way are the nurses and midwives. One in two staff fall into this category and there have been considerable debates around a simple question: should nurses be managed by other nurses or by general managers? As a largely female labour force, many nurses work part time and some work for one session a week or even less. Since the figures given above are for whole-time equivalents (WTE) the number of people involved is substantially greater. Regardless of who manages nurses, the management of a complex, differentiated labour force often providing a 24-hour service is a key management issue for the NHS.

Medical and dental staff   Medical and dental staff numbers increased by 16% over the period from 49 700 to 57 800. While remaining at about 5–6% of the directly employed workforce, they are a vitally important group who initiate and terminate a large proportion of NHS expenditure through direct decisions or through the consequence of decisions about whether to treat, investigate or admit.

From the beginning of the NHS doctors have held the right to be consulted about service management policies and other developments which influence their clinical work. Indeed a key condition in the bidding process for trust status was that prospective trusts could demonstrate appropriate patterns for the involvement of doctors in management. Government viewed such involvement as an essential sign of the management capability of a unit seeking the independence of trust status.

Conflicts with managers (handwritten margin note)

Clinical directorate structures and clinical budgeting processes are important mechanisms for integrating clinical and service management. Clinical staff do not regard themselves as employees to be managed and attempts to create such hierarchical structures are likely to result in serious conflicts.

Professional, technical and therapeutic staff

The increasing numbers of professional, technical and therapeutic staff can be partly explained by two important developments:

- Technological advances in imaging and specialist services required staff who could understand new hard technology, who could operate, maintain, calibrate, and interpret the resulting data.
- The ageing of the UK population increases the number of people requiring rehabilitation and care of chronic conditions by staff who have specialist expertise and can operate with limited, direct medical supervision.

Indeed this therapeutic requirement is heightened by the wish to help patients to pursue independent lives and receive their treatment in their homes or similar settings. There are also instances where the appointment of a psychologist might be seen to be a flexible and clear alternative to a psychiatrist with all that a medical appointment entails.

Administrative and clerical staff

The administrative and clerical label originates from the Whitley Council set up to negotiate on behalf of a wide range of staff. It would be misleading to conclude that between 1981 and 1991 there was a 23% increase in the number of managers, who now comprise 17% of the workforce. This category includes, unsurprisingly, clerks, secretaries, typists, machine operators, as well as catering workers, health care assistants and other support services. Indeed the figures for England show that the number of medical secretaries, regarded as critical to the smooth functioning of clinical services, rose from 5627 in 1984 to 9751 in 1990. The introduction of the internal market has changed the composition of this group, with increased requirements for financial, information management and data analysis staff.

Looking at the figures for England alone, the senior and junior administrative staff totalled 21 247 (WTE) in 1980 and had grown to 29 737 in 1988. During the period the number of clerical staff remained constant at about 50 000. Changes in the basis of definition influenced these figures as did a phenomenon known as 'incremental drift' (see Box 4.2).

Ancillary staff

The most dramatic change appears to have been in the numbers of ancillary staff which fell from 220 000 in 1981 to 115 000 in 1991, a fall of 48%. This is largely accounted for by the introduction of

Box 4.2
Incremental drift

> During periods of pay restraint one option open to managers who want to reward staff or make jobs appear more attractive in the market is to allow appeals for upgrading or to regrade jobs prior to recruitment. Thus the rate of pay increases while the job may remain objectively similar.
>
> In effect there is a process of inflation in job grades while the basic pay scales remain unchanged. This process is likely to have resulted in some staff crossing the boundaries between clerical and administrative scales and others moving from junior to senior administrative grades.
>
> At a senior level, ministers were reported to be very concerned during the process in which NHS trusts and purchasing agencies were being created that *people should not be paid more money for doing the same job* (Kember and MacPherson 1994, p. 251).

Competitive Tendering

competitive tendering arrangements instituted in 1983 for domestic, catering, and laundry services (DHSS, 1983). These services continued to be provided mostly by the same staff who were forced to accept new employers and often experienced reductions in their pay and conditions. Managers could not, however, contract out the responsibility for producing specifications for services, negotiating contracts, and ensuring compliance by the contractor. During this decade skills in the development, negotiation and management of contracts increased but not without some expensive mistakes on the way.

Costs

Hospital medical staff

A series of problems had to be faced relating to the numbers, grades, and specialisms of hospital medical staff. Increases in the numbers of medical students and changes towards equal numbers of male and female medical graduates began to cause difficulties in the career development process, with many registrars spending excessive times in training grades with little prospect of appointment to consultant status.

Shortages + Time Consuming

Additionally the NHS suffered from shortage specialties where the supply of specialist medical staff failed to keep up with demand, resulting in a rationing process and the need to seek approval for appointments. Government responded with plans to expand the numbers of consultant positions and to control the numbers of specialist training positions. (DHSS 1987).

GPs, dentists and optical practitioners

In 1981 there were 54 300 GPs, dentists and optical practitioners contracted to the NHS and by 1991 this figure had risen to 61 100 (UK figures). In England in 1990 there were 49 434 independent practitioners comprising 27 523 GPs (56%), 15 480 dentists (31%) and 6431 optical practitioners (31%). Over this period the average

Box 4.3
Gatekeepers to the
specialist services

GPs, dentists and optical practitioners play an important part in the NHS but are not direct employees. For many patients they are the first and only contact in a sickness episode. They act as gatekeepers to the specialist services and so their referral rates have an important bearing on the demand for hospital and community services.

It is often cheaper to manage sickness episodes in general practice than within the hospital services and patients often find the experience less intimidating. It follows that many recent policies have attempted to increase the range and complexity of cases dealt with in general practice. There is still much to learn about the outcomes of such practices for patients.

number of patients per GP has fallen from 2150 (1981) to 1900 (1991).

During this period there have been changes in the range of work undertaken by GPs and also in their views about the nature of services offered (see Box 4.3). Whitehouse in Chapter 6 shows that many GPs are undertaking minor surgery, while many GPs believe that it is no longer acceptable for them to be personally available 24 hours per day. There have been developments in deputizing services sometimes operating as collective arrangements by a number of local practices and in other cases as independent organizations selling their services to GPs. However such services are delivered, they are the subject of national contracts between the NHS and the GPs with local variations to take account of service requirements in an area 'managed' by the FHSA or, more often, by a combined purchasing authority.

It is important to note that while the GP's income is dominated by the contract for services it is not the only source of income. GPs are entitled to take private patients, to work for insurance companies, and to earn fees in other ways. Thus GPs may hold positions as clinical assistants in a specialist health care facility and be absent from their practice for one or more sessions per week. Frequently, any such appointment will be treated as partnership income and participation in any such employment will be a collective decision for the partnership. The GP contract goes so far as to set minimum training requirements for GPs to ensure that they are regularly updated on clinical and related developments.

As independent practitioners, GPs usually work in partnerships and are for all practical purposes small or medium sized businesses. They employ a variety of clinical, administrative, and managerial staff and frequently buy specialist skills on a fee-for-service basis. The GP contract and the local FHSA/Purchaser determine which staff are acceptable for salary reimbursement

GPs

PROFIT *SEEKING*

within the contract and what proportion of that salary will be reimbursed.

The GP partnership will be the leaders of a clinical team funded by a variety of arrangements. Some will work for the local community trust and have a base within the practice premises, others will be employed and funded entirely by the general practice as a business decision in which clinical and financial considerations are brought to bear. For instance, a practice manager might be appointed on administrative and financial grounds since such an appointment might be thought to increase practice efficiency or even practice income. Thus, GPs and their staff are increasingly expected to make similar decisions to those of any medium-sized business.

Other staff and volunteers

Finally, the workforce is supplemented by a wide variety of volunteers, employees of voluntary organizations, and carers who provide a significant proportion of the care but are not usually subject to the same incentives and other motivators which are thought to apply to employees. The effective use of such contributions requires understanding the special skills and expectations which volunteers bring to their work. Frequently the work done through voluntary organizations is subject to contracts, although those organizations are dependent on the willingness of their volunteers to comply with requirements. The positive side of this arrangement is that voluntary organizations may provide an inexpensive but good quality solution to some operational requirements of health services.

EXPECTATIONS AND CONSTRAINTS

E.U. Expectations Need to be taken into acc

All organizations must learn to live with the constraints imposed by scarcity of basic inputs – expertise, staff, revenue and capital availability, as well as paying attention to the external environment, markets and regulatory authorities. The NHS spends 20% of total government expenditure each year and is therefore never far from the centre of government attention. As employer of one million people it is a key part of the UK economy and also increasingly subject to the regulations and influence of the European Union. These regulations are designed to facilitate mobility of labour, encourage uniformly high standards of care, and increasingly meet the European conceptions of what it means to be a good employer. It follows that managers of clinical services are not able to act by paying sole attention to the requirements of a particular group of patients or services. Their hands are tied and they need to take account of a wide range of factors which may constrain their action.

Despite the internal market, the NHS remains firmly within government control and this has important implications for the management of both staff and contractors. It must provide a

*SElf
Referrel
Continues.*

comprehensive service, largely free at the point of need for all UK citizens and, through reciprocal arrangements, for EU citizens as well. It is not an option to exclude any but the most marginal services, although services previously provided by specialists are increasingly being provided within generalist settings, particularly primary care.

The 'right' of self-referral by attending an Accident and Emergency department means that many services must be a combination of elective work and responses to those who walk in through the door – even if a proportion of them are regarded as inappropriate or trivial attendances. Part of the service must operate 24 hours per day for 365 days per year. Demands for services cannot be entirely controlled and some staff will need to be available 24 hours per day.

Government, and indeed the population, demands a 'national' as well as a comprehensive service – implying similar quality and quantity of health care across the country. Measures to promote equity of provision include:

- the weighted capitation resource allocation formula;
- performance indicators;
- measures of levels of unmet need and waiting times;
- controls over the allocation of capital resources, especially buildings and large investments in technology.

The promotion of comprehensive, national and equitable services is intended to be met by government decisions about the top management structure of the service, including legislation on the broad pattern of board membership to be adopted by authorities and trusts. Gray and Jenkins in Chapter 1 point to the role of the Audit Commission in setting standards for public management and reviewing management practice in particular functions and locations, advising government and management on good practice.

The government has devised policies and programmes to improve the service to patients, as in the *Patient's Charter* (DoH 1992), and has set measurable objectives in the form of outcomes for selected services in *The Health of the Nation* (DoH 1990). It follows that clinical managers have to take notice of externally imposed objectives as well as those which pertain directly to the objectives of their department, trust or authority. Frequently financial inducements are used to further progress towards government objectives – such as the waiting list targets or services for AIDS patients. Many health promotion targets in primary care are necessarily accompanied by fee-for-service payments. As if this were not enough, government promises to use performance indicators in the form of league tables to identify especially good and poor performance.

Clinical managers will see many of these externally imposed objectives as opportunities to develop the skills of their staff, to

EXTERNAL CONSTRAINTS

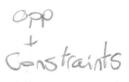

Opp
+
Constraints

increase the clinical capabilities of their department, or to increase the funding and perhaps the staffing of their department. Frequently constraints and opportunities come hand in hand and need to be recognized as such.

Shortfalls
in
Labour

EDUCATION AND RESEARCH

The NHS is an unusual organization since, in combination with the further and higher education sectors, it is responsible for funding and undertaking the initial and continuing education of most of its staff whether clinical or administrative. Consequently it has to match short-term requirements to balance its books, with longer-term requirements to secure an adequate labour force for the future. The failure to plan for future manpower needs results in unavailability of staff of the right calibre. In some cases the failure to undertake appropriate clinical manpower planning for the NHS has resulted in 'shortage specialties' and an inability to develop services at the required speed. Alternatively, the service is forced to find new ways of providing services without the skills that would have been desirable.

Coop
Consortia.

In the view of the government and the NHSE it should be the role of the employer to determine what patterns of training are required. In the case of the larger staff groups and of professional updating and training, employers are expected to form consortia who will purchase training from providers – which may be hospitals but will also include colleges and universities. Small groups of staff where there is only a limited demand are likely to be purchased by the centre, since the temptation not to invest in such areas is very real for a local provider, and there could be excessive costs in ensuring that local providers are coordinated into an appropriate purchasing arrangement.

In the light of the comment made above about the scarcity of finance to pay staff, it is an important and difficult question as to whether the labour force is likely to be large enough for the needs of the NHS in coming years and to what extent it will require to be extended through training mechanisms.

Box 4.4
Women and management in the NHS

The evidence of the existing patterns of management appointment are that in the past if you sought promotion from a clinical to a managerial position it helped to be male. The introduction of equal opportunities legislation has begun to change this particular bias and further instances of positive action such as Opportunity 2000 are designed to increase the proportion of women in senior management positions (NHSME 1992a). The NHSE has also created a Women's Unit which attempts to ensure that women appear on shortlists for interview for senior positions.

It is also unlikely that government will allow local employers to make key decisions on the numbers or types of place for medical training – whether for initial, specialist, or sub-specialist training. One key reason for this is that the Treasury regards doctors as a key source of expenditure and recent economic policies focus on the need to restrain public expenditure and where possible to cut it in absolute terms.

The NHS is also concerned with the development of specialist clinical and senior management staff most of whom are chosen from the ranks of clinical and administrative staff. Since the introduction of general management in 1985 the career progression of clinical staff within the NHS has altered. The introduction of clinical nurse specialists at about ward sister level created a specialist career option to contrast with the traditional routes of teaching and management. The abolition of District Management Teams meant that nurses no longer have a board position as of right and are frequently expected to hold a dual portfolio as nurse advisor and director of quality, consumer affairs etc. The opportunities for career progression for other staff have changed with the introduction of business manager or clinical nurse manager position within structures based on the clinical directorate.

The development and use of new patterns of management and organizational development using assessment, selection, and development centres have begun to replace the inequities of the appointment interview in which poor preparation by the appointments panel was often compounded by the lack of clear job and person specifications. While the interview has not entirely disappeared, its idiosyncrasies have been reduced by a wide range of **psychometric testing** accompanied by job sampling and other behavioural testing methods. These methods herald the shift towards a greater objectivity in the appointments process and point more closely to the capabilities of the individual and the requirements of the job. These technologies are also being used in developmental centres which aim to identify ambitious staff with above-average potential and to provide them with experience, secondment, training, and sometimes education programmes to prepare them to compete for top jobs.

It would be inaccurate to say that the NHS has adopted an enlightened human resources perspective in respect of all its staff, recognizing the organizational advantages of staff and management development and investing appropriately. There are still many 'black holes' where the only useful advice to an ambitious colleague would be to find another job quickly. Nevertheless the NHS is beginning to recognize that by investing in the development of its staff it may reap the reward of effective management and growing productivity – the investment may pay off although the harvest may be reaped by another employer at a later stage. It is still the case that investment in the discretionary development of staff is patchy and conflicts with other demands on scarce resources. Nonetheless there are many examples of good practice and ambitious staff are beginning to seek more than simply a job, salary and lease car.

Many doctors hold joint appointments with academic institutions as lecturers or professors and take part in a wide variety of research programmes, much training takes place on the ward, and patients are often involved in research programmes while they are being treated. The development of **ethical committees** is testimony to some of the problems which this entails, and auditors are increasingly interested in tracing the costs of research programmes and ensuring they are not inappropriately subsidized by service budgets.

Research plays an important role in most clinical settings, not least as an attempt to demonstrate the effectiveness or otherwise of clinical treatment regimes on services. Evidence of published research plays an important role in the clinical career progression of doctors seeking consultant appointments, as the pages of the *BMJ* or *Lancet* will testify. Increasingly, research is becoming a source of income for the NHS. Trusts may be keen to identify research opportunities and to harness the financial and broader benefits where it can be seen that the research is adequately funded and makes a clear contribution to the reputation and economy of the hospital. If, however, research is regarded as a drain on the funds available to fulfil service contracts then there is likely to be opposition to research programmes.

Contracts for research will be dependent on the pattern of services (and therefore the contracts for those services) of a particular trust. Recognition for training is also dependent on the pattern of services and the variety and volume of patients seen in a particular department. There is evidence to suggest that the quality of outcome for a patient is closely related to the number of patients seen and therefore to the collective experience of a department in dealing with particular problems. Indeed if this falls below agreed levels, recognition for training can be withdrawn, junior doctors will not apply for unrecognized appointments and services may have to be withdrawn.

Similarly, nurses in training still fill a significant proportion of the manpower requirements for the service and consequently their conditions of work and patterns of experience are expected to meet the expectations of the training authorities. Such conditions and the mechanisms for ensuring compliance are often set out in contracts of a similar pattern to service contracts. In the past decisions about training numbers were made at regional if not national levels and the issue for service managers was to understand the prevailing regulations and maximize the service contribution from staff in training. In today's NHS, service managers expect to determine future staffing requirements and enter into contracts with training providers, who are increasingly located in higher education establishments, to provide for their future manpower needs. *This highlights conflicts between short-term service needs and the use of resources to ensure availability of the right skills for the future.*

MANAGING PEOPLE IN THE INTERNAL MARKET

The introduction of the **internal market** has important implications for the management of staff. For ease of understanding we will consider the following categories:

- market managers;
- purchasers;
- providers and trusts;
- GPs and fundholders.

Market managers

Control

It was never intended that the NHS market should be cut free from its moorings and allowed to float unaided. The NHS regional health authorities played midwife in the setting up of trusts but the continuing role has been undertaken by 'outposts' of the NHSME. It is increasingly recognized that decisions with long-term consequences, such as closures, capital investments, and the development of centres of excellence involving the concentration of skills cannot be left to the local interests of the market or to the particular features of particular service contracts.

Purchasers

MANAGERS Decide which Role

outside consultants

The development of purchasing brought about the need for new skills and for existing skills to be brought together in new patterns and teams. Individuals who had previously been responsible for determining the pattern of services and for the line management of those services had to surrender one of their hats and become a purchaser or a provider. Managers who had previously been responsible for managing thousands of staff became responsible for tens of staff in new slimline authorities operating in a highly visible and uncertain context. Indeed the line-management skills on which many had built their careers became less important than analytical and planning skills directed to recognizing community needs for health care, contracting for services to meet those needs and monitoring provider compliance with those contracts.

The amalgamation of small purchasing units into consortia, followed by formal amalgamation and combination with FHSAs, widened the scope of purchasers to cover expanded territories, and to include primary, secondary and specialist services. Since they employed small numbers of staff, most purchasers could not justify employing dedicated Human Resource (HR) officers, although many called in such specialists to assist in the management of the change process and to help, often through consultancy arrangements, in the development of purchasing teams.

↓hrs
of Drs

H
O
L
D

C
O
N
T
R
A
C
T
S

F
I
X

W
A
G
E
S

M
E
A
N
S

O
F

F
R
E
D
U
C
I
N
G

C
O
S
T
S

NHS trusts   The foundation principle of trusts was that they were to be independent financial entities responsible for attracting business through a variety of contracts and for balancing income and expenditure. They were explicitly released from having to comply with the terms and conditions of national pay agreements negotiated through the Whitley Councils or by Independent Review Bodies. The major exception to this freedom was that they were bound to pursue the government's intention to cut the working hours of junior doctors to meet government pledges following widespread public disquiet. To some loud mutterings of disapproval they were to hold the contracts of all staff – including those of medical consultants which had previously been held by regional health authorities.

The new powers and freedoms opened a wide range of possibilities for trusts in their management practices and some parties expected them to be used. We shall look at some of the freedoms, the practical options open to trusts, and the ways in which they have, and have not, been employed.

Making decisions on broad employment patterns and policies

An increasing number of trusts are trying to address the broad question: what proportion of our revenue should we spend on the salaries, wages, and the associated employment costs of our staff? The Guys/St Thomas' trust was faced with the twin threats of **Tomlinson** and the reductions of contract income from many of its former 'customers' from outside central London (Tomlinson 1992). The view was taken that it would be desirable to reduce the percentage of revenue spent on staff from around 75–80% of total revenue to about 65–70%. By attempting to freeze new appointments, offering attractive severance payments, and more radical reviews of its staffing patterns, some progress was made but not without some local resistance from a range of interested parties. Many other trusts anticipating a shortfall in contract income, or looking to reduce their costs and so become more competitive in the market, have adopted similar policies – although these are not always made explicit for obvious reasons.

A more common process has been to adopt **incremental scrutinies**, skill-mix studies and job or work design analyses to address the issue in small steps. Thus decisions on new contracts, new categories of staff such as healthcare assistants, and even the attempts to identify the staffing requirements for new, adjusted services, provide opportunities for incremental adjustment to employment patterns while avoiding some of the resistance which might arise from addressing them directly.

For instance, the move to increase day surgery and the waiting-list initiatives require new patterns of service and therefore new patterns of staffing. More radical ideas include the use of hotel/

Box 4.5
The flexible
organization

> Various proponents of the flexible organization such as Charles Handy (Handy 1989) and Michael Cross (1985) have suggested that organizations will in future be composed of a small core group of highly skilled staff, and various forms of contractors who run particular services such as laundry, transport and catering, or who provide specialist skills when they are required (see also Atkinson 1985).
>
> The use of management and other forms of consultancy rather than inside employees, while not always successful, points to a concern to access scarce expertise and to be more cautious about the numbers of people who join the payroll. Such organizational forms allow the trust to focus on the needs of the core employees and to direct management and organizational development at this smaller group of staff. The performance of contractors is a matter for contract negotiation and management by core staff.

hostel style accommodation for some groups of patients with no more staffing than a similar hotel but with on-call arrangements as necessary. In such cases the HR policies adopted follow from the service strategies.

Choosing whom to employ

In labour intensive organizations it is vital that the experience, skills and knowledge of staff match the organizations' requirements, ensuring that particular staff are not over- or under-skilled for their role. The first situation results in inefficiency and the second in risks for the organization and its patients. Trusts were encouraged to examine ways of operating, for example through skill-mix studies, to find the optimum pattern of staffing and processes of working.

In practice this might mean the use of various **dependency models** to identify the right blend of experienced staff on particular wards using an objective assessment of the patients' needs. It might mean a different balance between highly qualified and less qualified staff such as healthcare assistants. It could certainly mean experimentation with the types of healthcare team used in different situations.

It became clear that if any staff had skills which became redundant due to changing circumstances of contracts, those staff, regardless of status, could be made redundant. In the past, making a consultant redundant had been considered virtually impossible without evidence of gross misconduct. In the market, if a trust fails to win a contract for a particular service then the specialist staff in that area are in danger of losing their jobs. However, such cavalier management can mean the loss of considerable skills and experience which the organization may not be able to replace in the future without incurring serious costs. It is always worthwhile investigating the possibilities of retraining staff with redundant skills to meet the new service requirements. This may have considerable benefits for the motivation of the whole group of staff and therefore for the performance of the organization.

Choosing the terms and conditions of employment

Different localities in the UK have different costs of living and property prices and consequently service managers may face more or less difficulty in filling a post and motivating the individual. The payment of a London allowance assumes that these costs should be recognized in pay formulae, and the per capita resource allocation process is designed to recognize the increased costs to employer and employees.

Where staff with particular skills or experience are scarce, managers face the dilemma of whether 'to make or buy', or in HR terms to train through an arrangement with a training provider or to buy through offering enhanced salaries or conditions. Existing staff may be happy to obtain new skills and training opportunities might be an important part of the motivation process. Alternatively, it may be simpler or cheaper to advertise for a particular skill and pay the required salary package.

In the past many NHS jobs were perceived as a job for life. This does not fit comfortably with the financial pressure felt by many trusts or with the standard duration of service contracts, some of which last for three years but many of which are annual. The introduction of 'senior manager' terms and conditions brought with it enhanced salary packages to reflect the valuation of the wider market but also included three-year rolling contracts, performance related pay, and contract extension related to satisfactory performance.

Given the powers to adjust salaries, terms and conditions to meet local circumstances, trusts have been reluctant to do so. Staff still expect some semblance of national comparability in their pay, terms and conditions and many trusts have been reluctant to step out of line. Local bargaining is a new concept for many NHS personnel and HR staff; and while many trusts have recruited such staff from outside the NHS, this does not mean that HR is a strongly managed discipline (NHSME 1992b). Fears of pay escalation are important and many managers see local pay bargaining as a can of worms (Seifert 1992). There is therefore a conflict of interest between the centre, the market managers, who would like to see the end of pay review bodies and Whitley Councils, and the trusts who perceive these bodies as a useful brake on wage pressure where a key local strategic objective is cost control.

RECOGNISE *COMPETENCIES*

Clones

Developing new patterns of management, organizational development, and training

Partly as a result of the development of new organizational forms, the NHS has begun to draw upon a battery of methods of organizational and management development in order to identify individual and group capabilities which can be linked to objectively identified organizational needs.

The creation of trusts led to new corporate and executive management roles and a variety of new 'technologies' were adopted to increase the likelihood of making good appointments. Once appointed, individuals and teams were expected to move quickly to high levels of performance; and so, on the basis of objective assessments of needs through assessment and development centres, personal development plans were adopted to encourage the rapid formation of high performing teams (see Box 4.6).

Box 4.6
Example

> South East Thames RHA and its constituent authorities and trusts set up a system to identify the broad competencies required of its 1000 top managers. These competencies formed the basis of development centres for managers who emerged with personal development plans and with some 'objective' evidence of their abilities, preferences, and areas in which development activities might benefit individual and organization. While such activities might be criticized for attempting to produce clones on the basis of the prejudices of existing managers, they did recognize that individuals have different preferences and abilities and their preferred methods of training and development benefit from an individualized approach rather than the application of a standard recipe.

Managing people in primary care

With the development of community care and of fundholding, and more generally the involvement of GPs in purchasing, the GP has had to pay more attention to the management of his or her practice staff. When compared with other providers general practices are of small size and require a measure of flexibility in the skills and the working practices of their staff.

The most obvious trend is in the development of the practice manager from a senior receptionist to a business manager, who in many cases acts as an informal partner. With the increasing complexity of data management and budgetary requirements, and with the gradual increase in average practice size, the practice manager needs to be an effective manager of people, many of whom will be part time and some of whom will be employed by a trust or will be a sessional employee of the practice.

MANAGING THE PERFORMANCE OF INDIVIDUALS AND TEAMS

Managing the performance of individuals and teams in the NHS is fraught with difficulties yet vitally important in the market context. Purchasers are charged with translating their revenue into the best possible package of care to meet local needs – in short they require value for money which puts pressure on providers to improve quality and to provide more care per pound. Renewal of existing contracts usually requires productivity improvements and so managers cannot avoid considering individual and group performance. The first difficulty is *measurement*.

The development of a wide range of **medical audit procedures** is intended to focus on the issue of clinical quality of work and to ensure uniformly high standards. Yet, perhaps inevitably so, this is an internal mechanism managed largely by those who are responsible for providing the service, in the first place.

A further issue in measuring and managing productivity revolves around **substitution** or the potential for substitution. We mentioned above that many tasks have been performed by staff who are primarily trainees – whether medical, nursing, or others. The so-called 'service contribution' of student nurses implies that less expensive staff with lower levels of certified knowledge, skills and experience might in some cases substitute for more qualified and hence expensive staff. This argument – and indeed the management practice which flows from it – has resulted in computer programs which claim to calculate the most cost-effective mix of staff in a given context. Such programs are, of course, only as good as the assumptions on which they are built and they soon lose credibility when clinical managers decide to use lower staffing ratios for financial or other reasons.

It follows that **productivity** can be improved:

- by increasing the output of a given group of staff;
- by using substitution to change the skill mix;
- by reducing related costs while maintaining or improving outputs.

Box 4.7
The difficulties of measurement

> It is relatively easy to count the number of patients seen in an outpatient clinic, but how do managers assess the outcome of these interactions? In another context, how might you compare the value of a 30-minute interview with a consultant or a similar interview with a specialist nurse which will usually have a significantly different cost to the provider organization. Is it acceptable simply to measure activity?
>
> An example of activity measurement is the 'consultant episode'. This measurement is used to provide a productivity measure for the NHS yet it has been criticized because it may be subject to double counting. It is certainly not clear that all consultant episodes are of equal value or cost.

Weigh Up Costs

COST TRANSFER OF JOBS

Reforms initially for Managers Later effecting Nurses Drs

These actions raise a series of thorny questions about *account-ability, risk, and the ethics of health provision.* Deciding whether a patient in general practice should be referred to a consultant psychiatrist, psychologist, counsellor, or not referred at all is a question to which significant costs may be attached. The GP's understanding of biomedical and behavioural science may compete with considerations of value for money and with the state of the practice budget and the nature of previous referrals.

So far our examples have focused on clinical work where decisions are regarded as being complex. There are, however, some complexities that result from new patterns of providing services. At a basic level the contracts for cleaning and domestic services often transfer operational management problems to out-side contractors and sometimes result in a lower bill for the hospital, but the experience varies. Sometimes the result is an inflexible service, domestic staff no longer find time in their new schedules to talk to patients, and variations to the contracted service prove expensive. With the 1994 decision of the European Court on the rights of staff when their employer changes being translated through the UK courts at the time of writing, the cost of this procedure of substitution may prove to be even higher than expected.

The **Griffiths reforms** brought with them an emphasis on the accountable individual, the person in charge, and related develop-ments included **individual performance appraisal** and **per-formance related pay**. These started as primarily managerial developments but clinical staff are increasingly being drawn in to such processes. In 1994 the BMA and the RCN came out publicly against proposals to introduce performance related pay for clinical and medical staff, using a variety of arguments which emphasize the elements of teamwork in clinical care, the dangers of introdu-cing factory methods to decisions about life and health, and the perverse effects on patient services of individual incentives and personal goals.

Since many services are provided by multi-disciplinary teams whose members are paid according to different scales, terms and conditions, the use of objectives, measurements and incentives poses a minefield for clinical managers. How, for instance, might you measure the contributions of the different staff who work in operating theatres? How can you justify the fact that some will receive overtime payments if a session overruns while others will not? Since each contribution, we assume, is necessary, can they be measured objectively? It has been more common to work with staff to try to assess what activities are required in particular work areas and then to assign an appropriate complement of staff. Of course changes such as the development of new anaesthetic and surgical techniques inevitably bring about changes, and these can be utilized to improve traditional staffing patterns and optimize the use of scarce human resources.

Performance incentives can be realized in ways other than by personal financial inducements. Where a work group is particularly efficient it is possible to reward them by passing on the savings they make, or a proportion of those savings, to developments in their particular area. Bad managers respond by penalizing them with higher workloads and more patients or by removing the savings of an efficient clinical area to bolster an inefficient department – resulting in demotivation all round.

Careful task analysis assesses the task to be undertaken, links the procedural technology with the pattern of skills and staffing in an attempt to improve the effectiveness and the efficiency of services. So, for example, the increased use of lasers, computers and scanners demands staff who can make safe and efficient use of machinery. Such staff may not fall conveniently into existing professional or employment categories and so there is a need for retraining, or new types of staff. For instance, in some places Operating Department Assistants (ODAs) developed new skills to deal with the electronic equipment in an operating theatre while nursing staff performed more traditional roles. This led to demands from ODAs for recognition in career structure and reward mechanisms.

MANAGING PEOPLE IN CHANGING SITUATIONS

The NHS has experienced a consistent stream of change since its inception but in the last two decades the pace and intensity seem to have increased. Externally imposed changes resulting from government policy and legislation include a number of adjustments to the management structure, attempts to change the pattern and use of resources, and straightforward policies to change the location and pattern of services such as those resulting from the Tomlinson Report. Changes have resulted from the development of new clinical technologies and from the aspirations and actions of those staff who control them. Changes are increasingly being implemented to meet the new 'business objectives' of trusts and purchasing authorities.

It follows that clinical managers responsible for the design and implementation of changes are often the object of changes being decided and implemented elsewhere. For instance, the closure of institutions for the mentally ill and mentally handicapped has meant that medical and other staff working in residential institutions have been forced to adopt new community-based patterns of working, with or without appropriate training. Changes in management patterns have meant that clinical staff are increasingly responsible, directly or indirectly, to general managers who may not have a clinical background. Some clinical staff, through choice or circumstances, have taken on roles such as clinical and medical director in which they must span the divide between clinicians and managers.

New patterns of management and control imply an active approach to budget management by clinical staff not previously expected to consider the costs of activities. Management tasks previously undertaken by specialist management accountants are the daily requirement of clinical managers who have had to learn by doing. Perhaps most widespread is the need to work to contracts which increasingly specify protocols for service quality and mechanisms for decisions which have expensive consequences.

At the individual level, the prospect of change may be perceived as threatening in a number of ways. The pattern of relationships with other staff and with patients may be threatened. New patterns of provision may be thought to imply risks to patients or patterns of work which are undesirable. For instance, the suggestion of a consultant trauma service may be seen to imply 24-hour working by staff who thought that their appointment as consultant had curtailed such expectations.

Change also threatens the efficiency of the organization. Existing patterns of activities have to be stopped and new patterns adopted, often implying a period of double running, and it is hoped that meantime the patient will experience a seamless service. Sometimes staff will resist change because they object to its content or to the way in which it is carried out. Indeed the standards and beliefs of staff are important factors which ensure that services operate at high levels of quality and efficiency. *Changes therefore need to be planned and managed since the effective operation of a complex service demands the goodwill, competence and cooperation of its staff.*

Unfortunately there are no universal recipes for successful organizational change and even the changes which are imposed through legislation or executive decision often require adjustment to meet local circumstances and resources. Donald Schon argues that organizations and their members fight to remain the same and that there is a 'conservative dynamic' within most organizations which has to be overcome (Schon 1971). The positive side of this dynamic is that it helps to maintain stability and predictability which are positive assets except during periods of change.

Lewin (1958) argues that successful change requires the unfreezing of current attitudes, systems and behaviour, implementation of the required change, and the successful refreezing of the new patterns of activity and the attitudes and behaviours which support it. It follows that change requires the development of organizational and personal capabilities, the appropriate timescales to allow change to take place, and frequently additional resources. These resources may take the form of external trainers or consultants who specialize in the change process.

Figure 4.2
Managing change for
competitive success:
the five central factors

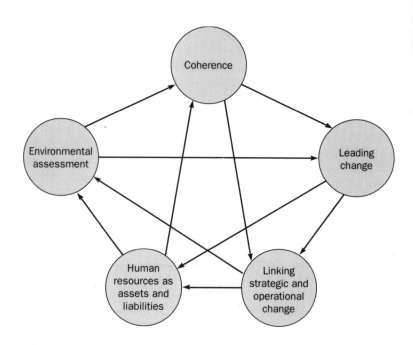

The chief exception to this process is where there is a real or artificial crisis. In the same way that private organizations facing a cash crisis take drastic surgery to ensure survival, so within the NHS the threat to the survival of a trust or hospital can be the spur to rapid and extensive change at organizational or individual levels. Essential lower-level objectives which normally take precedence are superseded by higher-level shared objectives which are usually unquestioned.

Pettigrew, Ferlie and McKee (1992), in their study of a variety of NHS changes, point to an important distinction between *receptive* and *non-receptive* contexts for change. Receptive contexts display the characteristics shown in Figure 4.2. Clinical managers need to develop and maintain receptive contexts which will increase the likelihood, but not guarantee, the effectiveness of attempts to change the patterns of activity within the organization.

SUMMARY

We have argued that the quality and responsiveness of clinical services depends on the effective management of people. This requires the balancing of immediate and future needs for staff and their skills within a context in which contracts for clinical services are the most important driving force. The introduction of the market has resulted in new roles and new freedoms and staff in post throughout the changes have had to learn new ways of working in situations of stress and uncertainty. In particular, new trusts must develop the skills to employ their freedoms without creating an escalation of costs through ineffective local negotiations.

As local services operating within a national health service there is an implicit conflict between local and national interests and short-term local considerations need to be matched against national requirements in the longer term. The competition between service providers may also need to be accompanied by cooperation to ensure that there is a capable and flexible workforce on which to draw in the future.

Finally, and perhaps most importantly, as the leaders in the development of new patterns of services, clinicians must pay careful attention to the development of the staff who will provide such services to ensure that quality is maintained.

FURTHER READING

◆ Journals: Human resource issues are dealt with in the *Health Service Journal* and the *NHS Manpower Review.*

◆ Handy, C. (1989), *The Age of Unreason,* Business Books, London.

◆ Kember, T. and MacPherson, G. (1994), *The NHS – A Kaleidoscope of Care,* Nuffield Provincial Hospitals Trust, London.

◆ Seifert, R. (1992), *Industrial Relations in the NHS,* Chapman & Hall, London.

REFERENCES

Atkinson, J. (1985), The changing corporation. In: Clutterbuck, D. (Ed.), *New Patterns of Work.* Aldershot: Gower.

Chief Medical Officers (1994), *A Policy Framework for Commissioning Cancer Services.* London: Department of Health.

Cm 555 (1989), *Working for Patients.* London: HMSO.

Cross, M. (1985), Flexible manning. In: Clutterbuck, D. (Ed.), *New Patterns of Work.* Aldershot: Gower.

Department of Health (1990), *The Heads of Agreement on Junior Doctors' Hours of Work.* London: HMSO.

Department of Health (1990), *The Health of the Nation: A Strategy for Health in England.* London: HMSO.

Department of Health (1994), *Health and Personal Social Service Statistics for England.* London: HMSO.

Department of Health (1992), *The Patient's Charter: Raising the Standard.* London: HMSO.

Department of Health and Social Security (1983), *Competitive Tendering in the Provision of Domestic, Catering and Laundry Services.* HC(83) 18.

Department of Health and Social Security (1987), *Hospital Medical Staffing: Achieving a Balance.* London: HMSO.

Griffiths, I. (1983), *NHS Management Inquiry.* London: HMSO.

Handy, C. (1989), *The Age of Unreason.* London: Business Books.

Kember, T. and MacPherson, G. (1994), Human resources. In: Kember, T. and MacPherson, G. (Eds), *The NHS – A Kaleidoscope of Care.* London: Nuffield Provincial Hospitals Trust.

Lewin, K. (1958), Group decisions and social change. In: Swanson, G. E. *et al*. (Eds), *Readings in Social Psychology.* Holt, Rhinehart & Winston: New York.

NHS Management Executive (1992a), *Women in the NHS: An Action Guide to the Opportunity 2000 Campaign.* London: Department of Health.

NHS Management Executive (1992b), *The Effectiveness of Personnel Management in the NHS,* (Riccardo and Peccei).

Pettigrew, A., Ferlie, E. and McKee, L. (1992), *Shaping Strategic Change.* London: Sage.

Schon, D. (1971), *Beyond the Stable State.* New York: Norton.

Seifert, R. (1992), *Industrial Relations in the NHS.* London: Chapman & Hall.

Tomlinson, B. (1992), *Report on the Enquiry into London's Health Service, Medical Education and Research.* London: HMSO.

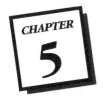

CHAPTER 5

QUALITY IN HEALTH CARE

**Barbara Morris
and Louise Bell**

OBJECTIVES

- ◆ To discuss the meaning of quality and how it might develop in the NHS.
- ◆ To explore and assess existing quality initiatives in the NHS.
- ◆ To see how the internal market might influence questions of service quality.

INTRODUCTION

The new-style National Health Service implicitly requires the inclusion of 'quality' in order to improve the effectiveness and efficiency of its services, and this emphasis is also evident in private sector health care. Yet, despite this common objective, there seem to be almost as many views about what quality is as there are professions in health care, and what is often perceived is a plethora of disconnected and sometimes conflicting initiatives – and all too often, patients see little or no improvement.

In this chapter we discuss the meaning of quality and outline its current and possible future perspectives in health services. Existing work in the health service and other associated fields will also be briefly explored and evaluated. The chapter will look at quality in the health service in light of the many recent reforms within the 'new market driven health arena' and discuss some of the implications of these reforms.

STIMULI FOR ACTION ON QUALITY

A number of general environmental influences on quality will be outlined later. First we look at several specific stimuli for attention to quality in the NHS.

Efficiency

The health service faces increasing demands created by innovations and developments that have led to the ability to treat more conditions, and by technology and improved environmental conditions that have led to increased longevity for the population. There have also been increases in the incidence of chronic, as opposed to acute diseases. While the costs of providing health services have gone up, often because of increased levels of technology, incoming resources have decreased because of unemployment and lower birth rates, which have reduced the total working population.

Much of the apparent never-ending demand for health care is related to the model of health care in use. This is very much a model of health as freedom from disease, and of health care as being focused on the treatment of disease. This model inevitably leads to increasing demand for health care for two reasons:

- An ageing population leads to an increase in chronic disease whilst 'uncorrected' habits associated with modern western-style living lead to an increase in some acute diseases, such as heart disease.
- Continuing medical research increases the range and scope of diseases which can be treated.

A different model of health as being a state of well-being would shift the focus to *prevention* of disease, and conceivably reduce demand, at least in areas such as coronary heart disease. In part, such a shift is indicated by the White Paper *The Health of the Nation* (DoH 1990b) which introduced targets for reducing the incidence of some diseases.

However, at least in the short term, health services are faced with increasing demand and constrained resources. This reinforces a need for quality in the sense of providing defect-free services and products, which are 'right first time' and do not involve the added expense of correcting things that have gone wrong.

Griffiths recommendations

The Griffiths recommendations (1983) placed quality on the management agenda. Throughout the 1980s there was considerable management-directed effort put into quality assurance, with much emphasis on standard-setting. The levels of commitment and effort devoted to this by the various professional groups varied considerably, but in the main, activities focused on separate aspects of the package of care provided to patients. Nurses, for example, developed nursing standards, whilst outpatient managers developed standards for non-clinical aspects of outpatient clinics.

The NHS review 1988

Further stimulus for quality came with ministerial review of the NHS in 1988. Two White Papers, *Working for Patients* and *Caring for People* placed emphasis on quality, amongst other issues. The ensuing 1990 legislation separated purchasers of health care from providers, and quality moved into the contracting arena. Providers increasingly recognized that quality was an issue on which they could differentiate themselves from competing providers, whilst purchasers became more conscious of the need to specify aspects of quality in the contracts they placed.

Department of Health initiatives

Yet further stimulus came from the Department of Health, which in the late 1980s funded demonstration sites to pilot the introduction of Total Quality Management within the NHS. (Total Quality Management is an organization-wide approach to quality. This will be discussed in more detail later.) A variety of projects ranging from quality assurance initiatives through to full Total Quality Management programmes received funding in 1989 and 1990.

District health authorities

DHAs were required to develop quality review procedures which covered a variety of aspects of quality, such as the reduction of waiting times, improved appointment systems, information to patients and the specification of quality elements in contracts.

Medical and clinical audit

Increasing attention was directed towards audit, particularly medical audit, and central funding was provided to encourage the setting up of appropriate audit procedures. The primary objective of such audit is peer review of the quality of treatment provided to patients.

Targeted activities

Some areas have been the subject of particular focus by the government. The initiative to reduce waiting lists is typical of these. Such initiatives have been narrowly focused on specific targets, and supported by additional funds.

All of the above have stimulated attention to quality, and a number of them are discussed in more detail later. However, whilst considerable action has been taken to encourage quality improvement, it is difficult to identify a clear picture of what quality is and how it should be managed. There is considerable imperative to focus on quality, and some clear indicators about particular aspects which should be given priority, but it does not constitute a coherent whole.

One can therefore say that there is no 'universal' definition of what quality is in health care, but that quality is a major issue. There are also difficulties with a 'universal' approach to quality in the NHS because it is a countrywide organization that has many sites, but is fragmented in nature and has differing local needs.

WHAT IS QUALITY IN HEALTH CARE?

At first glance this may seem to be a superfluous question, but in fact it is extremely difficult to define quality in exact terms because, like many aspects of the healthcare service, it seems to be nebulous. Another area that is similarly difficult to place into one concrete context are the many therapeutic interactions involved in a consultation. Yet despite the difficulty of exact definitions, everyone 'recognizes' quality when they see it!

The seductive nature of the quality message is such that the concept itself is open to abuse (West-Burnham 1992). No-one can overtly deny its importance – like motherhood and apple pie, quality is lauded. It is often seen as a panacea for problems affecting the organization, and public avowal of its importance supposedly reassures patients and other customers. However, in practical terms, the achievement of quality requires more than slogans. According to Juran (1980), quality does not just happen; it has to be planned.

The problem is that different people interpret and value the same experiences in different ways. What is 'quality' to one person may not be 'quality' to the next. For example, a nurse may regard each in-patient having a named nurse responsible for them in hospital as being good quality. The patient, on the other hand, may not agree; maybe he or she does not like that particular nurse, or feels that he or she cannot get attention from any other nurse (which, sadly, is sometimes the case). Often, different professionals involved in providing different aspects of the same service view quality in different ways, and this can cause conflict between people who are all dedicated to looking after the patient, but have different views about what he or she should receive. The definition which is adopted, implicitly or explicitly, in any situation, colours and directs the activities which people carry out. It is therefore important that in any situation all the people involved agree about what quality is.

Box 5.1 contains some definitions from a survey of health service staff from a variety of professions. These definitions indicate some of the general ambiguity about quality. One cause of ambiguity is that quality has connotations of both excellence and standards (Ellis 1993).

♦ If quality is *excellence*, as is its normal connotation in everyday use, then anything short of a Rolls Royce is clearly not good quality, and quality can only be aspired to by very few.

♦ However, if quality is something to do with *standards*, then it is far less abstract and is available to many. Quality in these terms exists when goods or services meet the specification laid down for them.

A second ambiguity, which is particularly acute in services provided by professionals or services that are purchased by someone other than the direct consumer, is the assumption of *who*

[handwritten margin note: DIFFERENCES OF OPINION(S)]

- 'A service I would be happy for my family to use at all levels'
- 'Audit'
- 'Conformance to requirements'
- 'Objective and systematic approach to improving care based on professional judgement, professionals set the lead'
- 'Quality is a subjective title given to a perceived degree of excellence in service provision'
- 'Value of something in terms of its success, acceptability and availability'
- 'Attaining professionally agreed standards of care'
- 'Something that is good, serves its purpose, and is worth the money that is paid for it'

judges the quality. The first of the definitions in Box 5.1 implies that quality is defined by what the writer thinks is appropriate for his or her family; the frame of reference is the family. The fourth definition, however, places judgement about what quality is firmly in the court of the professional, though without specifying _which_ professional, or what happens when professionals disagree. The third definition clearly has the connotation of quality as a standard, whilst the fifth equally has the connotation of excellence.

The _Collins Concise Dictionary_ in 1992 defined quality as

A distinguishing characteristic, the basic character or nature of a thing, a feature of personality.

This might be a useful everyday definition, but it is not particularly helpful for those trying to manage quality because it begs the question of what that 'distinguishing characteristic' is, and who determines it.

There are numerous definitions of quality that have their origins in industry, such as:

- 'Zero defects' (Crosby 1979);
- 'Fitness for use' (Juran 1979);
- 'Delighting the customer' (Peters and Austin 1985);
- 'A way of managing the organization' (Feigenbaum 1983).

Each of these represents a slightly different view of quality in terms of focus and strategy for managing it, but such short phrases cannot encompass the true nature of the views of quality taken by these authors. Juran (1988) himself counsels against using short phrases

Box 5.2
Quality – some
common themes

- ◆ Quality must be seen as a primary organizational goal, which includes all the functions in the organization.

- ◆ Quality is determined by the customers of the organization. Being aware of, and responsive to, customer requirements is integral to most ideas about quality, and this includes both internal customers within the organization who perform work or provide services for each other, as well as external customers.

- ◆ It is customer satisfaction which drives the organization because only by continuing to anticipate customers' requirements, and hence outstrip the competition, can organizations be successful.

- ◆ The study and reduction of variation in process is crucial because too much variation leads to a reduction in quality.

- ◆ Change is seen as being continuous and accomplished by teams and teamwork. The notion of continuous improvement is fundamental to most writers, and the complexity of most processes places them beyond the control of any one individual.

- ◆ Top management commitment is essential to promoting a culture of quality, for empowering employees to improve quality, and for the long-term perspective which is essential.

such as these, and emphasizes that it is important to take time to define the term. There are, however, some common themes among these writers which seem to be important (Melville 1994) and these are summarized in Box 5.2.

Whilst, conceptually, these commercial and manufacturing based ideas about quality can be transferred to the service sector, the literature generally suggests that because services are intangible in nature, service quality is more difficult to define. Additionally, only a very brief examination of the literature indicates that far more attention has been paid to quality of products than to quality of services. This is changing. The current and increasing number of service industries worldwide, concurrent with the decline in the manufacturing base, have all meant that research into service quality is widespread and increasing.

Research into quality in health care has often begun from first principles, but some workers in the field (e.g. Bell, Morris and Brown 1993) have begun to adapt work from the service industries' field and use it as the first step into establishing relevant issues in

Box 5.3
BS 5750

> BS 5750 is the British Standard for quality assurance systems. Its focus is the system which guarantees the quality of the service, rather than the service itself.

the NHS quality field. Others have examined approaches such as BS 5750 (see Box 5.3) which have their roots in manufacturing (e.g. Rooney 1989; Smith and Wain 1993).

It is important that rather than re-invent the wheel, a service such as the NHS examines relevant literature, tools and techniques from associated fields and uses these, rather than investing time and resources in unnecessary ventures. It is equally important, however, to recognize that the issue of defining, measuring, monitoring and improving the quality of health care has been addressed since time began. From Hippocrates through to Florence Nightingale, professional providers have been concerned with the quality of the care they deliver. However, the last ten years or so have seen a significant shift in the focus and emphasis on quality.

THE QUALITY IMPERATIVE

In the NHS, the advent of general management following the Griffiths recommendations (1983) brought a managerial focus on quality. The immediate post-Griffiths years saw the appointment of Quality Assurance managers, or similar posts. This can be seen as the first addition to the traditional professional role in quality management, with management being tasked with responsibilities for quality.

Whilst this was happening within the NHS, there was growing emphasis on the consumer in other sectors. This was driven by a number of strands. Perhaps the most powerful was direct consumer pressure, driven in part by increasing litigation, especially in the USA, for better standards and for a voice which product and service providers listened to. Another powerful pressure was competition. Major western industries, such as the car industry, were losing business to the Japanese, who had for years been improving the quality of their products. In the late 1970s and early 1980s quality became a major concern for both governments and industries. This was evidenced in Britain by quality initiatives from government, through the Department of Trade and Industry, and by actions taken by major companies such as Ford. In the business world in general, quality improvement became a major imperative, and increasingly, the customer became the driving force.

These external influences had an impact more widely on customer expectations of public services, which in turn has been felt by healthcare services. Customers have become more exacting and demanding, and this is evidenced by increasing challenge to clinical decisions (Moores 1989, Illich 1975).

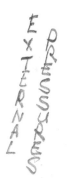
EXTERNAL PRESSURES

*Customers
No
Direct
Say.*

C
H
A
R
T
E
R

At the same time, government concerns for efficiency led to a series of measures, resulting in major moves to introduce a market economy model into the public sector. These have led to a partial, though many would argue, an imperfect, market model which tries to bring more competition, and by implication, more of a 'customer orientation' into the NHS. One key feature of this market model from a quality point of view is that patients are not the direct customers who purchase the services, *and there is considerable dilution of the direct consumer pressure*.

A second factor, perhaps at face value more influential than the market economy and efficiency measures, has been the political drive for quality. The Department of Trade and Industry was extremely influential in quality improvement in the British manufacturing sector, and then in business more widely, through a series of campaigns starting in the 1970s, with the current one being the *Managing in the '90s* programme (DTI 1992). Similar encouragement can be seen to come from Prime Minister John Major, who has established quality as a central element in public sector services, through the **Citizen's Charter** initiative. The Citizen's Charter sets out the principles of public service (see Box 5.4).

The net effect of these changes has been to introduce two further elements into the traditional notions of what quality is in health care: the importance of the customer or consumer, and value-for-money.

Despite this emphasis on the consumer and value-for-money, it is important not to lose sight of the fact that, in a professionally provided service such as health care, *there are some elements of the service that the consumer is not qualified to judge*. For example, few patients are able to judge the technical aspects of invasive surgery. However, there are problems with professional responsibility which it is equally important to recognize. Some

Box 5.4
The Principles of public service (Melville 1994)

♦ Explicit standards, published and prominently displayed at the point of delivery.

♦ Openness about costs, people and achievements.

♦ Information in comparable form, independently validated, to produce pressure to emulate the best.

♦ Choice, so that users' views are sought regularly and systematically to inform decision-making about services and standard-setting.

♦ Accessibility through flexible opening hours.

♦ A system of redress and a complaints system for when things go wrong.

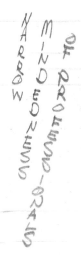

professionals take too narrow a view of the service, focusing only on the direct medical treatment of the condition, and failing to see that this is only part of the total service package; whilst some have too great a view of their professional expertise, and presume they always know better than the patient, and therefore should always make the decisions about what service or treatment is to be provided. This may be appropriate where there is no choice, but if choice is available, better professional quality may come from allowing the patient some say. Few patients could make a choice unaided between laparoscopic cholecystectomy, lithotripsy or traditional surgery for gall stone removal, but many of them would welcome knowing that there are alternative treatments, being able to discuss the pros and cons of each with the well-informed professional, and being able to express a preference.

TOWARDS A NEW DEFINITION OF QUALITY

When all the foregoing points have been considered, we have a view of quality as being concerned with satisfying professional views of what is appropriate but also being concerned with what customers want, and what represents good value in terms of the use of resources.

Box 5.5
BS 4778; Part 1, 1987

[Quality is the] totality of features and characteristics of a product or service that bear on its ability to satisfy stated or implied needs.

This leads to the adoption of a definition of quality which is based on the British Standard definition (Box 5.5), but incorporates the idea of value-for-money, and recognizes that the consumer of healthcare services is not necessarily the purchaser of them. Our definition is:

'Quality in health care is the total package of features and characteristics of a healthcare service or product, and the way in which it is provided, that bear on its ability to satisfy the agreed needs of the consumer and the agreed requirements of the purchaser within constraints imposed by professional judgement, at lowest cost, and whilst minimizing waste and losses.'

This is a long definition but incorporates a number of elements which we regard as fundamental to healthcare quality in the 1990s:

◆ *totality* of features of the product or service *and the way in which it is provided*: This recognizes that particularly for the consumer, and to a lesser extent the purchaser, quality is concerned with far more than the technical aspects of what is done or provided. It is also concerned with features such as timeliness, courtesy, choice and availability.

♦ *ability to satisfy needs of the consumer and requirements of the purchaser within constraints imposed by professional judgement*: This incorporates overt recognition of the fact that consumers and purchasers may have different needs and requirements, but that quality is judged primarily from their point of view, and not the provider's. Professional standards should not be contravened, but satisfaction of such standards is not sufficient to satisfy quality requirements.

♦ *at lowest cost*: this recognizes that value-for-money is an integral part of quality, and the cost of providing the product or service should be the minimum *compatible with meeting the requirements*.

♦ *whilst minimizing waste and losses*: This recognizes that waste in all its forms adds to cost, but that the cost of such waste is often sustained in a blanket overhead, and not attributed to the cost of a specific product or service.

Problems occur when attempting to create an exact definition of quality in the healthcare field because of the diverse nature of many of its services and the many different current approaches to quality in the health field. The definition given above adopts a proactive view of quality which is not found in all areas of the health service, or indeed, of commerce and industry. It incorporates a philosophy of quality as being primarily concerned with meeting customer requirements; this is rather more than being 'defect-free', and implies a continuing awareness of what customers want.

CURRENT QUALITY ACTIVITIES IN THE NHS

Several different approaches to managing quality can be identified in the National Health Service:

BS 5750

The NHS is a service industry with most of its workload consisting of face-to-face interactions between its customers and the service providers. Most of the direct work with patients in the NHS fits general notions about services, which are that input depends on the client, production and consumption take place at the same time, and the output is often intangible.

However, many staff within the healthcare field do not have direct dealings with patients, and some of them, particularly in the housekeeping and building support services, have operational tasks which are closer to manufacturing than to service. Laundries and building maintenance services, for example, have very tangible outputs. Many of these, together with those such as ambulance services, with clearly identified outputs, have adopted the BS 5750 approach of trying to ensure that they have systems which are capable of delivering their services reliably to the specification they have adopted. Some of these have been externally assessed, and certified as having achieved the BS 5750 standard.

Medical and clinical audit

Reforms?

Self-Regulation by Professionals

The medical and clinical professions believed for many years that because they were the groups who had greatest contact with service users they were primarily responsible for the quality of service. This view was reinforced by the appointments of the first quality managers. Many of these had been senior nurse managers, and in many areas the post of quality manager was combined with a director-level nursing post. Professionals and quality are often seen as synonymous, so for many years various groups of professionals were unquestioned about their activities. In keeping with their professional responsibilities, they were regarded as internally self-regulating. However, over the past few years, there has been a move away from ready acceptance of informal self-regulation to formal regulation which involves others.

Whilst auditing of medical care has always been carried out by the medical profession, until fairly recently this has been an internal issue. **Medical audit** is defined in the NHS Review White Paper (Cm 555, 1989)) as:

> 'the systematic, critical analysis of the quality of medical care, including the procedures used for diagnosis and treatment, the use of resources, and the resulting outcome and quality of life for the patient.'

This represents a departure from earlier forms. The substantive difference is the increasing emphasis on systematic procedures, and the requirement for these to be practised throughout the healthcare field. Both statutory audit requirements and the emphasis on systematized approaches are relatively new developments.

Reviews not the same

Pts views not voiced (enough)

Medical audit is an expected part of routine professional practice for all clinicians working in the NHS, and an organizational structure and sets of procedures have been rapidly developed, aided by financial support from the Department of Health (Moss 1992). A parallel development has been seen in **clinical audit**, which is audit in professions other than medicine. Although not so systematic or widespread, clinical audit is becoming an expected process amongst other professional groups (Goldstone and Doggett 1989).

The literature on medical audit is growing rapidly, and there is a wealth of material which discusses the process from a variety of different approaches (see for example Devlin 1990, Shaw 1989, Department of Health 1990a). Clinical audit is also being increasingly discussed in the literature, and suitable methodologies to implement audit are continuously being designed. Often the audit process is idiosyncratic, with many NHS trusts and hospitals having their own publications (see for example Frater 1992). This is creating an audit process which is not standardized, and which is often divorced from other quality initiatives.

Integral to almost all of the work reported in the literature is peer review, based on professional ideas of what quality is. The patient's view seems to be missing.

In some ways it can be argued that professional audit is limited because it involves peers assessing each other's activities. However, it is difficult to see how the purely technical element of the treatment provided can be assessed in any other way. Unfortunately, too often it is an after-the-event review, which detects problems only *after* they have occurred. Recent scandals documented in the UK press, such as people who were not cancer sufferers being treated for the disease because of an incorrect diagnosis, or the use of incorrect diagnostic procedures, have highlighted existent problems with the peer review system.

In addition, audit is limited because it focuses only on specific conditions, treatments and their outcomes, rather than on the total service package experienced by the patient.

Yet a further problem is overlaps and gaps in auditing as each professional group in a unit develops its own method of audit. There are some attempts to develop integrative audit, as for example in Sunderland Health Authority (Sharp and Kilvington 1993) but these are still not in common use.

In some areas, clinical and medical audit are being referred to jointly as 'clinical audit' and several regional health authorities now allocate funds equally to all types of audit. This can be seen as a way of placing equal value on all audit activities by allocating resources equitably. However, extra funds have been provided for the establishment of medical audit, and whilst it is currently widely practised, it may be that there will be some dilution when the additional funds cease.

Auditing processes within the NHS have grown around the practice of initially setting service standards and then measuring whether or not these are met. There has been rapid development of off-the-shelf instruments that purport to measure the quality of professional services, and increased use of existing audit tools, such as 'Monitor' (Goldstone and Doggett 1989), which is a tool for nurses.

Audit has often been seen as the main way in which professionals can assess the quality of the services they provide, but as has been discussed this is not necessarily the case. Professional audit usually addresses unidimensional issues of relevance to the particular profession, and as yet in some professions there is little evidence of significant impact on the outcomes of professional treatment. Indeed, Maynard (1991), discussing medical audit, argues that the audit systems themselves need auditing, and that alternative methods of changing medical practice need to be examined. In addition, professional audit fails to address overall quality needs organization-wide. It has an important part to play, but should not be left in isolation from other quality management activities, or regarded as all that is necessary.

Managers and quality

Managerial professions have also seen audit enter their workplace as the need to account for expenditure has increased. Managerial audit can be seen basically as an activity which looks at the way in which resources are allocated and whether 'value for money' as a result of expenditure was sufficient. There now exists an inherent and spoken need to establish what, where and why resources were spent. This has been reinforced by the activities of the **National Audit Office** and the **Audit Commission**. These have had considerable impact on the development of managing value-for-money in other public sectors (Burns 1992) and have begun to work with the NHS.

The effect of expenditure on health of the population as a whole is another issue which is currently being studied. This can be seen as the result of the NHS reforms which have been an attempt to introduce a more business-like approach into the health arena.

Tools have emerged which attempt to offer answers to the value-for-money issues. Accountants and health economists are for example becoming increasingly involved in this area. The development of the health market has meant that theoretically now it is possible to establish where resources are spent and on what. Looking at value-for-money conceptually has, however, raised issues relating to the need for accurate statistics and data relating to the activities of the health service.

Prior to the reforms the database relating to accurate cost information was extremely poor in the NHS. Staff usually did not know the cost of anything they used, which meant that sometimes expensive items were selected and used rather than cheaper equally effective alternatives. It is interesting to note that subsequent to the reforms, awareness of costs generally throughout the service has increased. In this way the reforms can be said to have created certain quality improvements in terms of the **efficiency** of the service.

A further managerial approach is that of **organizational audit**, which is focused on the acute sector. In the United Kingdom, organizational audit has been primarily pioneered by the King's Fund, based on the Australian model. The audit provides a useful assessment of organizational effectiveness in meeting nationally agreed standards, and a growing number of hospitals are participating (Pitt 1990). However, Ovretveit (1992) argues that such audit only demonstrates that the organization has met a particular set of standards in the past, and that therefore this approach does not assure high quality of health care.

*Individual
initiatives*

As well as the general approaches outlined above, there have been countless initiatives at individual department or service level. Categorizing these is impossible, and singling out individual ones as examples is difficult. However, the Association for Quality in Healthcare, in conjunction with the British Standards Institution, has for the past three years offered awards under the **Gold Award Scheme** for praiseworthy initiatives. Past award winners give some idea of the kinds of activity being carried out. These have included awards for centralized waiting list review, telephone response in general practice, regional standards for nursing services, and peer review in independent dental practice.

Comment

Apart from audit, which is practised nationally, most of the above activities are driven by individuals. Although the Welsh Office has adopted Total Quality Management as the approach to managing quality in the NHS in Wales, there seems to be little which can be regarded as a national strategy for quality. There is a lot of attention to quality in mission statements, and much exhortation to staff to deliver quality, but little underpinning which turns slogans and exhortations into practical results.

There are also some contradictions. The market model requires that providers be free to treat customers according to their own particular circumstances, yet there are *ad hoc* directives and instructions which run counter to local wishes and needs. A typical example of this is the policy on AIDS, which often places emphasis on this condition at the expense of other local needs. Much of this is the result of a market model which is still, relatively, in its infancy. Lovell (1992) has pointed out that the bureaucracy model of a civil service (which has many parallels in the 'unreformed' NHS, not all of which have been eliminated) is no longer appropriate if customers are to be treated according to their own needs in an efficient and effective manner. Speller and Ghobadian (1993a), discussing local authorities, and Lovell (1992) both note that there is evidence of resistance to the changes needed for effective quality management. Speller and Ghobadian (1993b) also refer to evidence found in local authorities of window dressing, a failure to focus on the customer, and unwillingness to adopt participative styles which combine strategic vision and grass roots involvement. Currently, there seems to be some indication of the same aspects in the NHS. It seems likely that this will decrease over time, but there does seem to be a reluctance or inability in some areas to move beyond the grand statements and slogans to planned and systematic action to improve quality.

*THE MISSING
QUALITY LINK*

One area has been neglected comparatively in the quality activities taking place in the NHS. This missing link is the customer (or patient). Despite the pressures for emphasis on the customer, there has been little formal work on quality from the patients' or purchaser's perspective.

'Delighting the customer' (Peters and Austin 1985) and other such phrases are frequently highlighted as being the most important aspect of quality services; but the professional and managerial approaches, which are currently the main techniques used in the NHS, do not approach the patients' viewpoint issue formally. Both approaches deal with quality *from their own perspective* and often fail to involve the service users, or to consider how users feel about the service.

The lack of the customer's view is at odds with the modern paradigm of quality in commerce and industry, which makes customer requirements a primary determinant of quality. It is clearly evidenced in the British Standard definition of quality referred to earlier, or more simply stated by Dale and Oakland (1991, p. 1) as 'meeting the customer requirements and current and future expectations'.

However, there is a major difficulty in health care with incorporating customer requirements. *This is the issue of who the customer is.* The customer role includes a number of elements which in health care are spread amongst a variety of different people. Normally, customers select (or in some cases, design) the service; they pay for it; they benefit from it; they participate in it. Patients clearly participate in and benefit from the service. They also pay for it, but not directly. They do not design it, and their element of choice is extremely limited. The economic power they would have in a commercial setting does not exist in the NHS because their 'right' to choose and pay for the services they want is exercised by purchasers, who buy services on their behalf.

The explicit aims of the health service reforms are to increase consumer choice and improve the quality of healthcare provision. However, since providers are dependent on purchasers for their business, it seems likely that they will seek to satisfy purchasers, rather than patients. This is mirrored to some extent in the private sector, where insurance companies are becoming more proactive in determining what the patient receives through the financial mechanism of what they will pay for. *Whilst this is not a problem if purchasers' and patients' views coincide, there is clearly a dilemma if the needs and priorities identified by purchasers differ significantly from those of patients.*

An approach based on Total Quality Management would regard purchasers as being responsible for ensuring that patients' needs are met, and indeed this seems to be implicit in the contractual relationships which now govern health care provided by the NHS. However, purchasers seem to be operating at a fairly macro level in terms of their contractual requirements. They tend to specify the types of treatment to be purchased, or the types of patients to be treated. Micro-level contractual stipulations about quality for individuals seem to be fairly limited, and to be based on the requirements of the Patient's Charter, rather than on direct knowledge of what their own local patients consider quality to be.

The creation of an environment where patient views/needs/wishes are an intrinsic part of service design and provision seems likely to become a major issue as the NHS struggles to become a more market-oriented and cost-effective service, with GP fundholders, purchasers and providers of health care services in competition not only with one another, but also with the private sector which is ever increasing in size. The dearth of information relating to patients' views, wishes and needs seems likely at this stage to become more central to the debate about health service quality and audit.

Pts views may materialise with the mkt

THE DIFFERENCE BETWEEN DESIGN QUALITY AND DELIVERY QUALITY

One useful way to approach the management of quality is to recognize the distinct difference between the quality of design and the quality of the delivery. A particular service may have a very high design quality, but be delivered badly, or conversely, may have a poor design quality, but be delivered superbly. For example, in one outpatient clinic it is intended that patients are seen at the time of their appointment, but overbooking results in appointments not being kept; in maternity services in one area a policy decision has been taken that delivery under water is not permitted at all, but normal deliveries are handled very well. For some patients, neither of these constitutes quality.

Design quality

The formal element of design quality (see Box 5.6) is managed in the NHS through contractual relationships. However, there is considerable informal negotiation about design quality in discussion with patients and their carers. There is also considerable scope for changing design quality within contractual specifications, if the desire exists. Such changes may be self-financing because they direct attention away from aspects which are over-specified from

Box 5.6
Design quality

> The design quality is the specification of what the product or service consists of. It is basically a description of all the elements which should be present, or in the words of our definition, a list of what constitutes the *total package of features and characteristics of the product or service and the way in which it is provided.* So, for example, the design specification for an outpatient clinic might include a statement of how a patient is to be treated at reception, how long he or she should reasonably be expected to wait, what information should be provided prior to the appointment, what the conditions in the waiting area should be, and so on.

lack of understanding

FAILURE TO IGNORE THE PATIENT

the patient's point of view, or may cost very little because they address issues which do not require extra resources.

Poor design quality can result from failure to identify what the total package consists of. This can arise because people do not understand what is valued by the customer or consumer, or because the specification does not take into account all the elements which are important to the user.

One of the primary reasons for this kind of situation arising is the *segmentation* of the package. For example, a wide variety of different professions are often involved in the provision of inpatient treatment: surgeons, anaesthetists, nurses, cleaners, physiotherapists, pharmacists, kitchen staff, laundry staff and so on. There is a tendency in health care for each of these different people to develop their own specification (often referred to as a standard) for the part of the service they provide. The problem is that the inpatient does not experience each of these elements as a distinctly separate aspect. He or she experiences that totality as the experience of being in hospital, and sometimes the sum of all these disparate parts does not add up to a coherent good-quality whole. Different professionals are not always aware of what other professionals need in order to be able to provide good design quality; sometimes things which are important to patients do not 'fit' within professional boundaries; sometimes professionals are not aware of what matters to the patient; sometimes even if they are aware, they do not feel it is their responsibility.

Another primary reason for poor design quality is lack of understanding of what quality means to the patient or purchaser. In an increasingly market-oriented service, understanding of the dimensions of quality and the integration of the separate responsibilities into a coherent whole is important. This requires both identification of what constitutes the total package, and the specification of what needs to be done or provided within the framework of the whole, and not as disparate functional or professional elements.

There is a lack of empirically grounded material about patients' views of what quality is. Most attempts to assess the patient's view have involved the use of **satisfaction surveys**, but whilst these indicate levels of satisfaction with a wide variety of issues, they provide little or no indication of whether or not these issues are important (Morris 1990).

A number of writers have stated dimensions which appear important (for example Maxwell 1984, 1992 and McNicol 1992), but whilst their arguments are intuitively appealing, there is little empirical evidence to support them. Studies have been carried out by some health authorities which did focus on what patients really care about, for example work in Trafford and Worthing (Centre for the Evaluation of Public Policy and Practice 1991), and in Kensington, Chelsea and Westminster Family Health Services Authority (Dennis 1991), but these have not been widely published. In addition, the emphasis has been placed on the *process* of finding out what patients want, rather than trying to produce a generalized list of features or a validated tool for measurement, such as has been provided by Parasuraman *et al.* (1988) for commercial services.

One study which attempted to identify a generalizable list of the dimensions which patients consider to be important was carried out in Southend Community Care Services NHS Trust (Bell *et al.* 1993). This produced results which correspond in part, but not completely, to the dimensions identified by Maxwell (1984, 1992) and Parasuraman *et al.* (1985, 1988). The six dimensions identified by Maxwell for health care are *accessibility, acceptability, appropriateness, equity, effectiveness, and efficiency.* Parasuraman and colleagues identified *tangibles, reliability, responsiveness, empathy and assurance.* The research findings in Southend are compatible with both of these, but with an added dimension of *privacy.*

These studies confound the commonly held view that, given the opportunity, patients will ask for the impossible. What was striking in the Southend study was how relatively modest were the things that patients considered to be important; for example:

♦ to be listened to and their views treated as important;
♦ not to be treated as half-witted because they were old;
♦ not to be made to feel they were a nuisance or a moaner;
♦ not being treated as if they and their time were unimportant or lacked value.

The key theme of the limited work which has been done on design quality in health care is that quality is multi-faceted and multi-dimensional. However, it does seem that, in common with the findings in commercial services, the most important dimension is *reliability.* Reliability is 'the ability to perform the promised service dependably and accurately' (Parasuraman *et al.* 1988, p. 23). It includes keeping appointments on time, not cancelling or changing appointments, and keeping accurate records. Specifications, therefore, should cover *all* of the dimensions, not just those related to the treatment of the waiting time.

Delivery quality Often what is intended to happen does not happen. This can occur for a number of reasons.

Inadequate resources

Sometimes the resources just do not exist to deliver the design quality. A simple, though staggering, example of this was seen by one of the authors. A contract specified that a particular service should be available within 24 hours, and the provider unit had

Box 5.7
Delivery quality

> The delivery quality is the extent to which what is done actually matches the specification.

accepted this contractual obligation. However, the service required a clinical consultant, and only one such consultant was available. Delivering the specification required the consultant to be available within 24 hours for 365 days of the year – which implies no holidays, no illness, no time for training and development. This is pushing commitment beyond the realms of reason!

Another reason for resource inadequacy is *inadequate training*. Considerable training is carried out in the NHS, but most of it is concerned with the technical aspects of the job. Training in interpersonal skills and customer awareness is fairly limited, yet both of these are important for service quality.

Inadequate specifications

Although considerable attention has been paid to standards in health care, there are still some areas where standards do not exist. More commonly, however, there are too many standards, and staff do not know where the priorities lie. Also, many of the standards which do exist are too general, and provide too little guidance for staff. Glib phrases like 'a high level of service' are used, without specifying what that means.

A significant issue is failure to communicate service standards. One of the authors was extremely surprised when working with a group of registrars to discover that most of them had never seen the contract for their service, and did not know to what they were contractually committed. In order to deliver quality, people need to know what quality is. Leaving them to form their own judgement is neither fair, nor controllable.

Finally, very few of the standards are linked to performance measurement, appraisal and reward systems. This diminishes their importance for staff, and leaves management without an important means of encouraging conformance to the standard.

Feedback on what is being achieved, and the ability to change

There are two equally important features here:

♦ Data collection is needed to find out what is happening.
♦ The people doing the work need the ability to make any changes required if the specification is not being met.

If people are to deliver quality, they need to know what is being achieved. Surveys can help here, as well as audit, performance monitoring, and analysis of performance indicators. However, **feedback**, without the ability to change, is guaranteed to create resistance and cynicism on the part of staff, and a significant reduction in the quality perceived by the patient. The very simple example in Box 5.8 illustrates this.

Box 5.8
Example

A patient had a problem which required regular visits to an outpatient clinic. The visits were normally two-weekly, to check on the progress of treatment, but during the period this had been varied on one or two occasions to suit either the need of the consultant or the need of the patient, this being agreed at the end of the consultation. On one occasion, the patient went to reception after the consultation to make the 'normal' appointment in two weeks' time. The clerk pointed out that the clinic was overbooked because the consultant was away the previous week. 'No problem', was the response, 'make it the week after'. This the clerk refused to do, saying that if the consultant said two weeks, two weeks it had to be. She also refused to check with the consultant that the suggested three weeks was, in fact, perfectly acceptable. The 'solution' offered was 'I will fit you in right at the start of the clinic, before the first appointment'. The patient, noticing that her name was added to several which preceded the 'first' appointment, thanked her lucky stars that she had been fitted in at the beginning, rather than the end!

This simple example demonstrates a number of important issues:

♦ The consultant did not know about the overbooking because no-one had told him about it (feedback).
♦ The clerk did not know how precise or otherwise was the instruction to come back in 2 weeks (specification).
♦ The clerk did not feel able to take any effective action (ability to make changes).

The net result was a patient who felt embarrassed at having raised the issue, but who knew that what had been arranged for her was unnecessary; a clerk who was upset by a patient she perceived as a nuisance; and continuation of a situation which would inevitably mean that appointment times could not be kept, hence causing poor quality for other patients.

MANAGING QUALITY

Managing quality in essence means ensuring that the design quality is appropriate, and that the delivery conforms to the specification. However, each of these can be done with differing degrees of proactivity.

The key issue in design quality is to understand the customer's perceptions, and this can be done in a number of ways (based on Zeithaml *et al.* 1990):

♦ monitoring and analysing complaints, and using them to identify and correct problems in the service process (not to allocate blame);

♦ comprehensive studies of purchasers' and patients' expectations (not satisfaction surveys);

♦ systematically researching the views of those who have contact with patients;

♦ use of patient panels, support organizations and Community Health Councils to provide a continuous source of information about patient expectations.

The first of these is a fairly reactive approach to design quality, whilst the other three are proactive. The reactive approach is probably the cheapest one to adopt, but its impact on design quality is very slow, and savings here may well be at the expense of custom. Ideally, all four techniques will be used.

We now consider three basic types of approach to managing conformance.

Quality control   This is a fairly traditional approach which is based on the fundamental assumption that errors and defects are inevitable. This being so, the way to manage quality is to inspect or check after the event to make sure that things have been done correctly, and if not, to correct them.

In manufacturing, this approach works reasonably well in terms of its outcome, because defective products are detected and weeded out before the customer receives them. However, it is wasteful, because time, effort and resources are expended producing the items incorrectly in the first place, and having to correct them. There are also occasions when errors slip past the inspectors, and customers receive defective goods. It has limited use in healthcare services because by their very nature it is impossible to inspect any service involving the patient before he or she receives it. Hence any errors made are experienced directly by the patient – with sometimes disastrous and very costly results.

In methods designed purely to weed out defects or errors, there is no ongoing reduction in the number of defects or errors; this will only occur if information about the errors is passed back into a system designed to use them to improve the methods by which goods are produced or services delivered. This completion of the cycle by using the results of detection is vital if improvement is to be achieved.

Typical techniques included in this approach are sampling of the service or product whilst it is being produced, checking after the event through audit and survey work, and analysis of complaints.

Quality assurance   The quality assurance approach is rather more proactive than quality control. The basic assumption is that errors and defects are *not* inevitable. They can be prevented by systematic activity designed to ensure that the right result is achieved every time. Attention switches from inspection of the product or service in order to detect errors, to control of the inputs and the process by which products are made, or services delivered. The aim is to make sure that the inputs are correct, and the process itself carried out correctly. If both of these occur, the end result must be correct.

Methods of controlling inputs include careful specification of the skills required to do the work and appropriate training, and ensuring the quality of any materials used, either by quality control methods, or by pushing responsibility for ensuring quality back to the suppliers.

Processes are controlled by automatic control methods where appropriate (normally this only applies to machines) or by **statistical process control** (SPC). SPC is designed to enable the people doing the job to be responsible for its quality. To do this, they need to know whether the process itself is capable of meeting the requirements and whether it *is* meeting the requirements at any point in time. They must be able to make adjustments to either the process itself or to the inputs when necessary.

The most commonly used technique is a control chart. This is based on the normal variability to be expected from the process. So, for example, if patients in a GP's surgery are normally seen within 10 minutes of their appointment time, the normal variation is 20 minutes (10 minutes before time, and 10 minutes after). With this information, it is possible to construct a chart which can provide a warning when the normal variation changes. This change can only happen if something else has changed, either one of the inputs, or the process itself. The warning indicates when adjustments are necessary. Small samples are taken at intervals, and the results plotted on the chart. In effect, the control chart acts like a traffic signal, giving a red light when action is necessary, and staying at green otherwise. This technique has been used within health care, for example, to control infection rates, but is not yet common.

Often, quality assurance incorporates quality control techniques for checking purposes.

Total Quality Management

Total Quality Management (TQM) is much broader based, and much more proactive, than the other two approaches. Both quality control and quality assurance aim to meet the specification, and so they are focused solely on conformance. TQM goes a step further. Conformance is important but only as a step along the way. *The philosophy of TQM is that what is good enough today will not be good enough tomorrow, and so continual improvement is the aim.*

The initial step is to ensure that the existing requirements can be met every time, which in itself is often a major task. Once that is achieved, the next step is to improve the specification. Both quality control and quality assurance tend to treat the specification as given; their focus is meeting it. TQM incorporates the specification itself within quality management; its fundamental objective is satisfying (or delighting) the customer. The specification is not an end in itself – it is only the means by which customer requirements are described.

TQM often incorporates quality assurance, and to a far less extent, quality control, but is much broader in its approach than either of them. Both quality control and quality assurance deal only with the processes by which products are made, or services produced. TQM embraces the whole organization. The justification for this is that whilst many departments in an organization do not deal directly with customers, failures or errors there will sooner or later affect customer service directly, or indirectly by preventing some other department doing its job correctly.

For example, misfiling of a patient's record may create problems for a doctor and affect the quality of a consultation, or inadequate accounting procedures may lead to a department unwittingly overspending during the early part of a year, and having to cut back at the expense of patients during the later part.

Hence TQM embraces all departments in an organization-wide approach with the common objective of satisfying the customer. Because of this it requires high commitment from senior management to drive and coordinate it. Both quality control and quality assurance can be used in a piecemeal way, for example at department level, and controlled and managed at a fairly low level. The minimum appropriate site for TQM is a self-contained unit, such as hospital or a health centre.

A piecemeal approach to TQM is pointless, because sooner or later departments trying to practise it will come up against the resistance of those who are not, and who are not necessarily committed to the same objective of satisfying the customer. Additionally, piecemeal adoption of TQM can fail because organizational controls are not compatible. If the aim is customer satisfaction, measures of its achievement are needed, and care is needed to ensure that other measures or objectives do not conflict with this.

For example, if customer satisfaction is the aim, using control mechanisms focused on resource utilization may not be appropriate. Often the best way of fully utilizing expensive hospital equipment is to have a queue of patients, so that the equipment is not left idle. However, this would conflict with patient requirements for limited waiting, and the keeping of appointment times.

Of the three approaches to conformance, TQM is by far the most wide-reaching, and the one which is most closely linked to design quality. However, it is possibly too ambitious an approach for many healthcare sites at present. It seems to be most successful in situations where quality control and quality assurance techniques are already well-established.

SUMMARY

This has been a very wide-ranging chapter, touching on many topics related to quality, and demonstrating that quality is an integral part of health care. It cannot be hived-off as something separate, which is not part of everything from day-to-day activities right through to strategies for gaining or placing contracts.

Compared with industry and commerce, a few years ago the NHS was fairly naive in its thinking about quality. Much has been achieved in those few years, largely by the efforts of dedicated enthusiasts. It now needs to be grounded much more in the operating policies and activities so that the piecemeal development seen so far can become much more coordinated and coherent. In particular, much more attention needs to be given to the patient's view. Current services literature (for example, Mastenbroek 1991) indicates that in order for services to be successful in an increasingly competitive arena they must provide sufficient quality and meet customer requirements.

In order to meet the requirements of customers the NHS needs to alter its philosophy in terms of increasing its awareness of the views of patients and encompassing these into quality specifications and audit, and more generally incorporating them into the overall philosophy within the service. In terms of the creation of market forces, imperfect though they may be, it becomes increasingly important that those involved in the provision of health care services to consumers of those services – patients – provide a service that is 'patient friendly'.

FURTHER READING

- ♦ Journals: Up-to-date contributions can be found in the *International Journal of Health Care Quality Assurance*.

- ♦ Centre for the Evaluation of Public Policy and Practice (1991), *Evaluation of Total Quality Management Projects in the National Health Service*, Brunel University, London.

- ♦ Juran, J.M. (1988), *Juran on Planning for Quality*, Free Press, New York.

- ♦ Ovretveit, J. (1992), *Health Service Quality*, Blackwell, Oxford.

REFERENCES

Bell, L. and Morris, B. (1993), Patient-defined Audit. In: Johnston, R. and Slack, N. (Eds), *Proceedings of the OMAUK Conference*, Warwick.

Bell, L., Morris, B. and Brown, R. (1993), Devising a multidisciplinary audit tool, *International Journal of Health Care Quality Assurance*, 6(4).

British Standards Institution (1987), *BS 4778: Quality Vocabulary; Part 1, International Terms; Part 2, National Terms*.

Burns, T. (1992), Researching customer service in the public sector, *Journal of the Market Research Society*, 34(1).

Centre for the Evaluation of Public Policy and Practice (1991), *Evaluation of Total Quality Management Projects in the National Health Service:*

First Interim Report to the Department of Health. London: Brunel University.

Cm 555 (1989), *Working for Patients*. London: HMSO.

Crosby, P. (1979), *Quality is Free*. New York: McGraw-Hill.

Dale, B. and Oakland, J. (1991), *Quality Improvement Through Standards*. Cheltenham: Stanley Thornes.

Dennis, N. (1991), *Ask the Patient: New Approaches to Consumer Feedback in General Practice*. College of Health in conjunction with Kensington, Chelsea & Westminster Family Health Services Authority.

Department of Health (1990a), *The Quality of Medical Care*, Report of the Standing Medical Advisory Council. London: DoH.

Department of Health (1990b), *The Health of the Nation: A Strategy for Health in England*. London: DoH.

Department of Trade and Industry (1992), *Managing in the 90s: The Competitive Response*. London: DTI.

Devlin, B. (1990), Audit and the quality of care, *Annals of the Royal College of Surgeons* (Suppl), 72(7): 3-13.

Ellis, R. (1993), *Quality Assurance for University Teaching*. Milton Keynes: Open University Press.

Feigenbaum, A. (1983), *Total Quality Control*. New York: McGraw-Hill.

Frater, A. (1992), *Medical Audit in NW Thames*. London: NW Thames Regional Health Authority.

Goldstone, L. and Doggett, D. (1989), *Monitor*. Leeds: Leeds Polytechnic Enterprises.

Griffiths, D. (1983), *Report on National Health Service Management*. London: DHSS.

Illich, I. (1975), *Medical Nemesis*. London: Calder and Boyars.

Juran, J.M. (1979), *Quality Control Handbook*, 3rd edn. New York: McGraw-Hill.

Juran, J.M. (1980), *Quality Planning and Analysis*. New York: McGraw-Hill.

Juran, J.M. (1988), *Juran on Planning for Quality*. New York: Free Press.

Lovell, R. (1992), Citizen's Charter: the cultural challenge, *Public Administration*, 70:395-404.

Mastenbroek, W. (Ed.) (1991), *Managing for Quality in the Service Sector*. Oxford: Blackwell Business.

Maxwell, R. (1984), Quality assessment in health, *British Medical Journal*, 288: 1470-72.

Maxwell, R. (1992), Dimensions of quality revisited: from thought to action, *Quality in Healthcare*, 1:173.

Maynard, A. (1991), Auditing audit from an 'Ivory Tower', *Health and Social Services Journal*, 18(7).

McNicol, M. (1992), Achieving quality improvement by structured patient management, *Quality in Healthcare* (Suppl), 1(3): 40-41.

Melville, R. (1994), *An Assessment of Service Quality in a Higher Education College Registry*. MBA dissertation, Canterbury Business School.

Moores, B. (1989), The need for medical audit, *Medicare Journal of Management*, 3(4).

Morris, B. (1990), Incorporating customer requirements in health care. Presented at a conference on Total Quality Management in Health Care, Birmingham, October 1990.

Moss, F. (1992), Achieving quality in hospital practice, *Quality in Healthcare*, 1:17–19.

Ovretveit, J. (1992), *Health Service Quality.* Oxford: Blackwell.

Parasuraman, A., Zeithaml, V. and Berry, L. (1985), A conceptual model of service quality and its implications for future research, *Journal of Marketing*, 49.

Parasuraman, A., Zeithaml, V. and Berry, L. (1988), SERVQUAL: a multiple-item scale for measuring consumer perception of service quality, *Journal of Retailing*, 64(1).

Peters, T. and Austin, N. (1985), *A Passion for Excellence.* London: Fontana/Collins.

Pitt, C. (1990), Organisational audit: a national approach to setting and monitoring standards, *International Journal of Health Care Quality Assurance*, 3(3).

Rooney, M. (1989), *A Quality Management System for the NHS and a Strategy for Training.* NHS Training Authority.

Sharp T. and Kilvington, J. (1993), Towards integrative audit: a partnership for quality, *International Journal of Health Care Quality Assurance*, 6(4).

Shaw, C. (1989), *Medical Audit: A Hospital Handbook.* London: King's Fund.

Smith, J. and Wain, M. (1993), QUDOS: a quality assurance system for health care, *International Journal of Health Care Quality Assurance*, 6(4).

Speller, S. and Ghobadian, A. (1993a), Change for the public sector, *Managing Service Quality*, July, 29–32.

Speller, S. and Ghobadian, A. (1993b), Change for the public sector, *Managing Service Quality*, Sept., 29–34.

West-Burnham, J. (1992), *Managing Quality in Schools.* Harlow: Longman.

Zeithaml, V., Parasuraman, A. and Berry, L. (1990), *Delivering Service Quality.* New York: Free Press/Macmillan.

SECTION III

MANAGING KEY SERVICES

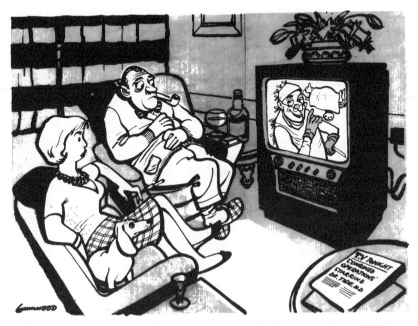

"Remember folks – for the cleanest cut of all – ring Doctor Tide – Harley Street 1212."

(First published in the *Sunday Dispatch*, 24 April 1960)

Patients do not come in homogeneous categories with discrete symptoms and clear diagnoses. Rather they have a wide variety of problems and frequently require services from a range of practitioners operating in different settings.

A particular episode of sickness may require services from family, GP, hospital specialist, and community care agencies, but not necessarily in that order. The management of a chronic disease may require a combination of these services over a period of years. While it suits our purposes to examine healthcare services in discrete categories, each of the authors is at pains to show how their particular service is connected to the others and how good quality services require the integration of a variety of institutions and practitioners.

We suggested in the Introduction that effective clinical managers require a deep understanding of the context in which they work and of the individual and collective capabilities which make up those institutions. Lengthy periods of specialist training tend to create professionals who are highly skilled in a narrow field of competence. Increasingly, clinical managers need a strong appreciation of the nature and contribution of complementary services provided by their colleagues since they will want to be able to provide patients with packages of care which meet their needs in a cost-effective fashion. This argument holds up to some extent within institutional forms and to a greater extent when we look across institutional boundaries.

The internal market is designed to create a series of incentives for providers to be more efficient in the production of quality services. This implies a pressure to identify alternative packages of care which will be provided by a number of agencies, and being able to identify the most cost-effective alternative. This will require good quality assessment of patient needs so that the best package of care can be constructed. Indeed some providers will identify the quality of their patient assessment skills as one of the strong features which distinguish them from other providers.

Within the market some GPs will be both purchasers and providers. They will be faced with the option of buying in a service or obtaining the resources with which to provide that service themselves. When they choose to buy or to refer, they will have clear views about what they require, ranging from what constitutes an appropriate waiting period to what they expect of the service to whom the patient has been referred.

Ideas about the role of different parts of the healthcare system are changing along with many of the underlying technologies. The development of non-invasive surgical techniques has changed views about the balance of inpatient and short-stay surgery, and purchaser and provider institutions consequently make different choices about investments, contracts and service developments.

Increasingly patients also have a clear view about what they expect from medical services. They expect to be involved in decisions which affect them, ranging from issues of convenience to questions of risk and treatment choice.

Carl Whitehouse writes as a practising GP and illustrates the remarkable changes in the pattern of services provided within primary care and the management difficulties which have resulted. From a position of relative obscurity in the profession the general practitioner has become a powerful purchaser of services and could in coming years be the largest purchaser in most localities. Since the purchaser will determine the shape of services and their particular form and content, all clinical managers are going to have a particular interest in the views of GPs and in the patterns of thinking and practice which evolve over the next few years.

Martin Knapp and **Robyn Lawson** approach their subject from the perspective of researchers with long experience in the development of policies of community care and their implementation. Many early assumptions portrayed community care as the cheap alternative and as a means of ensuring that expensive hospital beds were not taken by patients who could equally well be cared for elsewhere. As is the case with many important policies, the reality proved more complex than the vision and the management problems posed by the need to coordinate a large variety of providers were serious. Government responded in the form of legislation and other policy initiatives which are described in some detail, as are the management dilemmas and solutions which have been implemented by a variety of agencies.

Technology developments alongside changes in our understanding of the role of acute care and the interrelationships of various acute institutional types have changed the pattern of acute care and this has provided a series of problems for clinical managers. Government has attempted to shape the form of hospital services through the pattern of institutional development and through the management of the clinical, and particularly the consultant, staff, who largely determine them.

For many years the patient has been expected to defer to medical opinion in matters of treatment and the pattern of service provided and has been represented by largely toothless watchdogs. The advent of consumerism in the wider society associated with the ideas of the Citizen's Charter has placed the consumer on the agenda of every management board, but how can the diverse and sometimes conflicting views of consumers be represented without adding to the cost of services or to what is thought by many to be already an over-bureaucratic service? Do the various attempts to provide a voice for consumers add to the quality of services or to the outcomes or benefits experienced by patients? **Michael Calnan** reviews this important and difficult area, pointing to the main considerations for managers of clinical services and the main benefits to be achieved in this particular field of management.

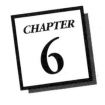

GENERAL PRACTICE AND PRIMARY HEALTHCARE SERVICES

Carl R. Whitehouse

OBJECTIVES

♦ To examine the implications of first-contact care.

♦ To explore the provider role of the GP.

♦ To identify the place of the patient in primary care.

♦ To evaluate the impact of health promotion requirements on the management of the general practice.

♦ To assess the purchasing role of the GP.

♦ To examine the management and monitoring of primary care services.

INTRODUCTION

Primary healthcare services provided by family doctors, dentists, community pharmacists, opticians and community nurses are central to health policy in the UK. The 1987 White Paper, *Promoting Better Health*, said that their importance cannot be overstated. General practice, therefore, has a key position within the NHS.

The implementation of the White Papers *Promoting Better Health* and *Working for Patients* through the 1990 Contract for General Practitioners and the NHS and Community Care Act 1990 produced a number of changes in these services. They were intended to provide patients with both better health care and better choice and to give greater satisfaction and rewards for those working in the NHS who successfully responded to local needs and preferences. The government stated these would:

♦ ensure the patient's requirements are met;
♦ raise standards of care;
♦ encourage health promotion and prevention of ill-health;
♦ increase competition and give the public a greater choice;

♦ improve service provision in inner cities and other deprived areas;

♦ improve value for money.

To achieve these aims required different approaches. Patients were to be provided with more information. Terms of service were to be changed to reflect what the government saw as good general practice (such as health promotion advice and improved availability of doctors). Remuneration was to be changed to become more performance related. Above all there would be greater emphasis on quality standards and audit.

This chapter focuses on general medical services and considers how the reforms have changed the traditional roles of these. We will see how these changes relate to the objective of providing high-quality accessible care. We will also consider the effects on other sectors of the health service and how it relates to the idea of purchasing health care in a community-based needs-oriented way.

FIRST CONTACT WITH HEALTH SERVICES

On an average day in 1990, 750 000 people consulted their family doctor. This is a rise of over a third since the mid 1970s. All age groups consulted more except men between 16 and 44. The average person now visits their doctor five times a year and half of these consultations are for new episodes of illness. In comparison the average person only attends a hospital accident and emergency department for a new episode once in four years. It follows that family doctor services provide the usual first point of contact for advice or treatment. The average doctor sees 35 patients a day, and sometimes twice that number, each with different needs. How do doctors make sure patients can see them with sufficient time to deal with these needs? Over the years this has changed (see Boxes 6.1 and 6.2).

In the 1950s general practice was a largely one-man (sic) cottage industry. Half the practices employed no administrative help and the control of accessibility and workload was entirely in the hands of the doctor. The seminal survey 'Good General Practice' (Taylor 1954) encouraged the development of administrative and nursing

Box 6.1
The way it was

'When I visited my doctor as a child, I went down to a large corner house in the suburb in which we lived, and crept in the back door where there was a cramped waiting area. A group of sullen-looking people sat round the walls eyeing each other to make sure no one jumped the queue. Every few minutes the doctor's cheery face would pop round the door and say "Next please". You would enter his warm room with its large desk and filing cabinet, and after the consultation was over would be let out by a french window.'

Box 6.2
The way it is

'When I visit my doctor today, I telephone to make an appointment. I am often told that the doctor is full for two or three days ahead, although I may see an assistant earlier if it is urgent. If I suggest it is urgent the receptionist will ask me what the problem is, and will decide whether to tell me to come down straight away, or book me in to the next available surgery. The receptionist may even offer me an appointment with "our practice nurse". When I reach the large but pleasant health centre it is crowded with patients waiting for six doctors. I have to wait for a buzzer to tell me when to go down the corridor. After my appointment I have to walk back to the desk, and make a further appointment with a practice nurse for some tests to be done, because the doctor did not have time to carry them out within the consultation.'

support in practices and the 1966 Charter provided resources for this.

Today, many people are involved in providing an accessible service. The general practitioner needs time for tasks other than face-to-face contact. The 1990 contract recognized this but did insist that patients needed to know when they could see their doctors. Terms of service were changed to make sure that a full-time general practitioner was clearly available for at least 26 hours a week, over five working days, at times convenient to their patients. But we need to look at other ways in which an accessible modern service is organized.

The receptionist

The key person in patient access to care is often the receptionist. Receptionists are much maligned, yet they play a critical role in the running of the practice and require very careful recruitment, training and support.

Appointment systems

Appointment systems were seen as a major advance years ago. Taylor (1954) commented that waiting at the surgery had become part of the British way of life, adding:

'The appalling waste of patients' time in doctors' waiting-rooms is a serious blot on NHS practice. Each year it must run into many millions of hours, representing a substantial loss in national production.'

He advocated the adoption of appointment systems, but noted the reluctance of doctors. He also made the comment that new appointments 'can seldom be made more than twenty-four hours ahead. Most new patients have complaints of fairly sudden onset, or more long-standing troubles where courage has to be screwed up. In either case, the need is for an immediate consultation.'

What is it like years on? The advantages of appointment systems to doctors in managing the flow of work are clear, but patients often find them a barrier rather than a time saver. Systems need constant review to ensure that there are enough spaces for people to have that 'immediate consultation'. Many practices have even reverted to partial appointment systems with some open surgeries.

The telephone and the nurse

The telephone rather than the counter is often the first point of contact with general practitioner services. Many patients feel their problem could be resolved without attending the surgery if they had the opportunity to talk to a doctor or nurse. It has been shown that patients appreciate telephone access (Hallam 1993) but in many practices they find the system deficient. This is a growing demand which requires skilled organization.

Some practices give nurses a key role in this, although the use of practice nurses (or nurse practitioners with an even more extended role) to provide first clinical contact with patients is still an open question.

Out-of-hours demand

Distress and fear caused by the onset of sickness are no respecters of time and out-of-hours cover is required. Traditionally this was provided by one's personal doctor, even if this meant being called away from a theatre or playing field. This personal responsibility remains a key feature of British general practice to which the public and government seem wedded. In the 1990 contract, for instance, the possibility of opting out was removed.

Doctors are responsible for their patients at all times, but anyone who has requested an out-of-hours call knows that you seldom see your own doctor at night and at weekends. Doctors share or delegate their responsibility through the use of rotas, cooperatives or commercial deputizing services.

A recent survey of general practitioners (Electoral Reform Ballot Services 1992) showed that most general practitioners consider that 24-hour responsibility is now outdated, and negotiations are taking place to end it. How will such care be provided in the future? Hallam (1994) found a number of approaches were being tried:

- a rota of general practitioners in a single practice or neighbouring practices;
- a cooperative of general practitioners covering a geographical area;
- a commercial deputizing service;

◆ a primary care emergency clinic;

◆ hospital accident and emergency department, possibly with employed general practitioners;

◆ a separate emergency medical service based on ambulances.

In these ways out-of-hours cover may become easier to access but less personal. What happens in the day will continue to influence out-of-hours care. If doctors are not easily available in normal working hours more people are likely to call out of hours, whilst the treatment of patients out of hours benefits from some understanding of their continuing needs.

First-contact care

Contact with the health services no longer resembles a trip to the corner shop. Although the organization is complex, failure to provide good first-contact care is one of the commonest reasons for complaint. In the light of this GPs have to solve the (management) problems identified in Box 6.3.

Box 6.3
Key management
issues for GPs

◆ How to balance easy availability with the need to plan appointments, clinics and time off

◆ How to ensure that the person with whom the patient first comes into contact has the necessary training and support to deal with people under stress

◆ How to provide a communication network that provides all first-contact workers with the information they need to help patients

THE GENERAL PRACTITIONER AS PROVIDER

Once patients have made contact with the doctor they expect some service. The idea of a general practitioner as a doctor with a pad of prescriptions, a pad of sickness certificates and a pile of referral forms was always a parody. General practitioners always provided a wide range of help for serious and chronic illness. Recent developments and technological advances have increased or altered this range of provision and a number of factors now affect the service a particular practice can provide:

◆ the range of skills possessed by doctor(s);
◆ the number and range of staff that can be employed;
◆ the available time;
◆ the number of potential recipients of service;
◆ the facilities and equipment available on premises.

A major factor in increasing the range of skills and staff has been the development of **group practice**. Over 20% of practices consist of six or more partners. Single-handed practices still exist but now account for only 10%. Smaller practices, of course, may extend their services by sharing premises or by being involved in fund-holding cooperatives.

The recent reforms have also affected service provision and we will consider four aspects:

- providing financial encouragement to carry out minor surgery;
- encouraging (through the health promotion initiatives) special services for the management of chronic illnesses such as diabetes and asthma;
- allowing greater variability in the range of staff employed by general practitioners;
- fundholding provisions that have enabled general practitioners to purchase services on or near their premises, including (since 1993) community nursing services.

Minor surgery   In different circumstances 40 years ago minor surgery was being given up by general practitioners (Taylor 1954). Taylor felt that, in most instances, hospitals were a better place for such activity. Improved premises, disposable sterile supplies, better local anaesthesia and the availability of practice nurses has changed this situation. Many general practitioners can again be involved in surgical procedures and a financial incentive was provided by the 1990 Contract.

Minor surgery sessions in practices can provide a faster and more convenient service for patients and reduce pressure on hospitals, but only if the following conditions are fulfilled:

- There is adequate training of the operator. The contract itself provides a list of procedures a general practitioner should be qualified to carry out. The **FHSA** minor surgery committee has to approve the skills, but criteria are not always easy to set.
- There are adequate premises and facilities. Again criteria for these should be set by the FHSA and are easier to standardize.
- Full resuscitation facilities are available *and* personnel are trained in their use.
- There is planned time for sessions with availability of support staff.

In summary, GPs need training, time and facilities.

Chronic disease   In the past the care of many patients with chronic conditions was
management   shared between hospital outpatient departments and the general practitioner. The hospital provided monitoring (such as regular investigations and consultation with other team members) less easily accessible in general practice. However, this led to *fragmentation of care* which was not always good for the patient.

Box 6.4
The diabetic mini-clinic

> Consider a 60-year-old female patient with diabetes controlled by tablets. She used to go to the local hospital diabetic clinic every 3 months for blood tests and examination, and then she had to go to her own doctor to get the tablets. Two years ago the practice started its own mini-clinic. It is run by one of the partners (not her own doctor) and a practice nurse. The local chiropodist attends, a local optometrist has checked her eyes and twice there has been a dietician there to talk about diet. She knows the diabetic specialist nurse from the hospital came to train the practice nurses, and the doctor has been on a special course – but she is not sure the doctor is as good as a 'specialist' and she sees her own family doctor less often.

Now patients are increasingly being encouraged to consider the practice as the appropriate place for monitoring their care. The diabetic mini-clinic (Box 6.4) provides an example of this new approach and its consequences.

There are several advantages to this approach:

- Patients can have most of their care at the practice premises.
- Special clinic sessions provide more time for examinations, investigations and discussions.
- Doctors and nurses develop special skills which increase effectiveness in advice, management and early recognition of complications.
- Patients can have easy access to other professionals.

There are also some disadvantages:

- Patients have less freedom in the time and place they can attend for care. The special clinics for individual conditions may be held comparatively infrequently (e.g. monthly) and at inconvenient times for some patients.
- Other doctors in the practice lose their skills and confidence in managing a common condition.
- The 'clinic' doctor may not be the patient's personal doctor and may be unaware of other factors affecting patients or their families.

This highlights the constant tension between providing personal care adapted to the individual and providing clinically skilled care. As more and more areas are retrieved by general practice this will be an increasing problem. No general practitioner can be a jack-of-all-specialties and practices designate one partner as their 'diabetes' expert, one as the 'asthma' expert, one as their 'surgeon' and so on.

The team approach also impacts on the traditional picture of general practice. As practice nurses become increasingly skilled, they are clearly (and rightly) seen by patients as practitioners in their own right. This gives patients a greater choice of key workers in a practice. They will often relate more to a 'diabetes nurse' or an 'asthma nurse' than to their own doctor. Patients will have different preferences, which will affect their choice of practice. Some will prefer the personal care of one doctor with a small support team in a single-handed practice, accepting that this may require referral outside the practice when the skills range is not adequate. Other patients may be less concerned to see the same person on each occasion and will prefer the wider range of skills in a large 'primary care centre'.

Increased range of skilled staff

Before 1990, FHSAs could reimburse general practitioners 70% of the cost of employing nurses, secretaries and receptionists, but *not* counsellors or computer clerks. The reforms removed the bar on the range of staff for whom general practitioners could be reimbursed. At the same time funding changed so that FHSAs were no longer committed to 70% reimbursement for every eligible post. The money could now be deployed in ways that reflected local priorities; for instance some areas used it to encourage the employment of practice nurses. This greater flexibility has also been used in more innovative ways. General practitioners have sought funding to bring a range of skills such as physiotherapy, dietetics, psychology and counselling into their practices (see Box 6.5).

The patient in Box 6.5 might wonder if it is better to see a counsellor, and this example identifies some of the considerations in assessing such developments in general practice. Attitudes to mental health have changed frequently. Taylor (1954) is instructive when he states: 'It is a surprise to find ... how comparatively seldom

Box 6.5
The practice counsellor

Ten years ago Mr Wilson had a 'breakdown' and went to see his doctor. The doctor gave him some tranquillizers and also saw him at the end of surgery for four or five weeks for some long chats which helped him sort out his problems. Recently he has been going through another difficult time and went to see his new doctor who seemed reluctant to use any form of tablets. In the end he came away with some 'antidepressants' and an appointment to see the practice counsellor who, he was told, was very good at helping people talk through their problems. He was not sure about keeping the appointment but in the end he did. He found the counsellor very understanding. It was helpful, and he knew he was not holding his doctor up.

the good general practitioner diagnoses neurotic illness'. He later says that: 'Claims that as many as a third of the general practitioners' patients are suffering from neurotic illness appear to have arisen mainly because organic complaints have not been diagnosed'.

Language and attitudes have changed. 'Neurosis' now seldom appears in general practice language and since 1954 we have seen the 'Rise and Fall of the Benzodiazepines' as managements for anxiety-related symptoms. Today, on the one hand, GPs are being asked to be more aware of 'depression', especially when it may respond to antidepressants. On the other hand, as drug treatments are seen to have their own dangers, a number of new approaches are being developed to help people. Some of these are psychological such as behavioural relaxation techniques and a range of counselling approaches. A third of general practices in England and Wales now have counsellors, but it has been reported (Sibbald *et al.* 1993) that many of these lack qualifications and are referred problems outside their knowledge. Wiltshire FHSA carried out an audit in their own area (Wiles and Macalister Smith 1993) and found that general practitioners were not always aware what counsellors could do, there was poor communication between counsellors, practice staff and other services and there was a lack of consensus on outcomes. This led them to set strict criteria for funding counsellors:

◆ Counsellors should work at a level equivalent to the British Association of Counselling accreditation.
◆ Counsellors should have a least 300 hours of direct counselling experience.
◆ Counsellors should have an explicit arrangement for supervision.

Different Therapies

The foregoing example shows how unproven new ideas can be taken up enthusiastically when they seem to offer an answer to a difficult and distressing problem. Attempts to limit development to interventions which have proven results fall on deaf ears when people are trying to care in situations of distress and breakdown. For many reasons, including the move towards community care of the mentally ill, general practice is having to deal with more psychological problems. Physical distress and immobility brought on by joint and bone conditions can produce similar problems. People want to try physical therapy techniques or complementary medicine approaches even if they are unproven. Ascertaining what skills will best benefit patients is a difficult task in general practice.

Increasing services on premises   Fundholding has encouraged many general practitioners to consider what resources they need to purchase from outside the practice, and what might be more economically and efficiently provided within the practice. Minor surgery has already been

Box 6.6
The Desktop Analyser

> A typical GP has had a number of patients requesting a cholesterol test. For some time there have been conflicting reports as to the value of the test, and who should have it done. There are also differing opinions on what should be done if a raised cholesterol is found. However the local pharmacy has recently introduced a service for testing and some patients seem surprised that their doctor is not doing the same. She is considering the purchase of a Desktop Analyser but is still troubled by a number of questions about accuracy, cost and legal responsibility if the practice provides tests. If people are found to have high cholesterol further investigation and treatment might increase hospital and practice workload without much evidence of worthwhile outcomes.

discussed, but there are many other possible investigations and treatments. The dilemma described in Box 6.6 is a good example of the issues affecting introduction of *new technology*.

British general practice has long been an art with minimal technology. This is one reason for its comparatively low cost in marked contrast to the primary care services in many other countries. Moving some investigatory work to general practice may be seen as a way to reduce overall costs. This is not necessarily true. In a recent study of the introduction of what is termed **near-patient testing** for standard investigations in general practice, no evidence of cost-effectiveness was found with the exception of midstream urine analysis (Rink *et al.* 1993). GPs must be aware that they risk incurring greatly increased investigation costs. Four questions therefore need to be asked prior to introduction of any test:

- Is the test likely to alter management?
- Is the test reliable and accurate?
- Is the test required with reasonable frequency?
- Is the test equipment easy to maintain?

The most difficult, and arguably the most important, is the first.

Comment   The four developments discussed above pose important issues if general practice is to provide more effective primary care. Many innovations have been introduced as much on enthusiasm as evidence. Enthusiasm encourages innovation. It is less good for effective and economic development.

Some innovations have been responsive to patient demand. This is an encouraging sign, but is not a good reason for ill-considered developments. Patients can, and will, change their mind if it is found that the service they demanded is, in reality, more uncomfortable or even more dangerous than what it has replaced. With this in mind GPs will wish to consider the following questions:

- What evidence is being presented that a new provision will be effective?
- What evidence is there that patients want the new provision?
- What facilities, equipment, staff and training will be required?
- How much extra time will the new provision need?
- Will the new provision mean that there is less time and money for a well-tried and valued aspect of general practice care?

PUTTING PATIENTS FIRST IN PRIMARY CARE

Central to the stated strategy of the NHS reforms has been the extension of **patient choice**. This is explored further in Chapter 9, but a number of strategies proposed to achieve it in primary care will be considered in this section:

- improved choice of general practitioner;
- the Patient's Charter;
- patient participation groups;
- the general practitioner as gatekeeper and bridge-builder.

Improved choice of general practitioner

A market-oriented approach to health care implies increased competition between general practitioners. Two small reforms were essential:

- The first was to make it easier for patients to change their general practitioner.
- The second was to allow general practitioners to tell prospective patients what services they offered.

Before 1990 a patient who had not moved address but wished to change general practitioner had to seek their previous doctor's consent or go through a complex procedure of giving notice to the FHSA. This has changed so that patients are able to ask any other general practitioner to register them. General practitioners are still free to decide whether to register the patient or not. Since many practices will not take transfers, it is not clear how much increase in mobility of patients has followed the reform.

But how can patients decide on a doctor? They need *information*. This can be found in the **medical list** and in **practice leaflets**.

The 'medical list' (a directory of local doctors) used to contain only a brief statement of qualifications and other services (such as obstetric care or family planning) provided by the doctor. The prospective patient will now find details of times of availability, languages spoken, clinical interests, access for the disabled, and staff details.

More important in providing information for the patients was the

Box 6.7
The practice leaflet

As well as the information in the medical list, this must include details about:

♦ use of appointment systems and means of obtaining non-urgent and urgent appointments

♦ the provision of clinics

♦ methods of obtaining non-urgent and urgent domiciliary visits

♦ whether the doctor works single-handed or in a group, and whether part-time, etc.

♦ arrangements for providing services when not personally available

♦ repeat prescription systems

♦ staff who assist the doctor in practice, including details of any assistants and whether the practice is a training practice.

♦ the geographical boundary of the practice area (with a map)

♦ arrangements for receiving patients' comments on provision of general medical services.

change in the doctors' terms of service to require compilation of a practice leaflet (see Box 6.7).

Such leaflets, to be supplied to every patient on the list, encourage informed choice but the details may not be easy to assess. For instance a large practice will specify a wide range of clinics for different conditions, whereas a single-handed practitioner may provide exactly the same services within routine appointments. Holding diabetic clinics or antenatal clinics is only of value if there are enough patients who would choose to attend at a given time, and sufficient staff to organize and run the clinics. Patients should not be misled into a belief that the presence of a particular clinic means a better service.

The Patient's Charter

Following the implementation of the GPs Contract the government introduced its **Citizen's Charter** initiative. The **Patient's Charter** reaffirmed seven well-established rights, and introduced three new ones as from 1 April 1992. The established rights were to:

♦ receive health care on the basis of clinical need, regardless of ability to pay;

♦ be registered with a general practitioner;

- receive emergency medical care (through general practitioner, ambulance or A&E departments);
- be referred to an acceptable consultant 'when your general practitioner thinks it necessary';
- be given a clear explanation of any proposed treatment;
- have access to health records;
- choose whether one wishes to take part in medical research or medical student training.

All of these relate to primary care, as do the new rights to an efficient complaints procedure and to detailed information on local health services including quality standards and maximum waiting times.

FHSAs were given local charter standards from November 1992, and the Patient's Charter for Family Doctor Services in March 1993 encouraged practices to produce their own standards. The proposed standards were set out in the 1992 Circular ((EL92)88 Annex D) starting with the words

'We are committed to giving you the best possible service. This will be achieved by working together. Help us to help you.'

This concept of partnership, and of patients' rights being balanced by patient responsibilities, has been taken up in a number of practices. One single-handed practice in a difficult inner city area (Moss Side, Manchester) has developed such a charter and found it acceptable to patients and staff alike (see Box 6.8).

Box 6.8
A local charter

> The Charter provides details such as how soon appointments can be expected, and the statement that patients will always know to whom they are speaking when they telephone or visit the surgery. It talks about respect for the patients' privacy and dignity. It also includes a section on patient obligations such as requesting repeat prescriptions in good time or not smoking in clinical or waiting areas. It balances statements that the staff will be courteous and friendly, with an expectation that patients will treat receptionists in the same way.
>
> (D. Shlosberg and J. Shlosberg, personal communication)

Patient participation groups   Many years before the charter initiative some doctors had developed the concept of partnership through **patient participation groups**. Peter Pritchard (1994) has been a key figure in these developments and lists possible activities as follows:

♦ reconciliation of patients' goals with those of doctors and staff;

♦ providing feedback for evaluating existing services and future planning;

♦ ensuring care for under-served groups in the community;

♦ linking primary health care with other community services;

♦ helping to develop effective prevention and promotion programmes;

♦ influencing other organizations in order to bring about change;

♦ a forum for complaints and suggestions;

♦ supporting the work of the practice (e.g. newsletters and equipment).

He points out that such partnership implies a well-integrated team in an effective and participative organization which requires investment in the management infrastructure.

Referrals –
gatekeeper or
bridge-builder

The medical etiquette for many years, reinforced by the new purchaser–provider situation, means that patients cannot usually see a consultant without a referral from a general practitioner. This restrictive, or gatekeeping, role is considered important in keeping down the cost of British health care. It was confirmed in *Working for Patients* which said

'The general practitioner – acting on behalf of patients – is the gatekeeper to the NHS as a whole.'

The only major hospital units with open access are Accident & Emergency Departments and Genitourinary Medicine Clinics (for sexually transmitted diseases).

Fundholding has even decreased referrals between departments within hospitals. A patient attending an Accident & Emergency Department for a non-traumatic condition will no longer be referred on for an orthopaedic or ENT appointment without the prior agreement of the general practitioner. The general practitioner becomes the key adviser, best qualified to advise whether or not someone needs to go to hospital, which hospitals offer the best service, and who are the best specialists to consult.

How does this role relate to patient choice? In one survey of attitudes to the referral process (Mahon, Wilkin and Whitehouse 1994) only half of general practitioners thought it appropriate often or always to give patients a choice of hospital, and only one in ten patients reported being offered a choice of hospital by their general practitioner. One factor in this failure to offer much choice may have been the paucity of information on which to base advice. Half the doctors did not receive any information about waiting lists from outside their own district (Mahon *et al.* 1993). There is even less information available on clinical outcomes (see Box 6.9).

No rational choice can be made by general practitioner or patient without better information on the options. The ideal situation may

Box 6.9
The patient with
cataracts

> Mrs Kinnock has recently been found to have cataracts. She knows that the waiting list at the local eye hospital is very long. She has friends in a major centre 75 miles away and wonders if she should go there. This poses problems for the general practitioner. It would be an extracontractual referral for which this year's budget has run out. The general practitioner has no information about the current waiting list at the distant hospital, or about the success and complication rates of the two hospitals.

GP as

Bridge builder

rather than

Gate keeper

be for the general practitioner to become less a gatekeeper than a bridge-builder. As a bridge-builder the general practitioner will help the patient's choice by providing and explaining information. Once the mutual decision about a referral is made, the bridge-builder will facilitate the links with the hospitals. Hospitals increasingly perform only part of the investigations or treatment, with patients returning to the community for care by the primary healthcare team. The general practitioner needs to explain what might happen, respond to the patient's choice and then negotiate and build bridges for the patient to pass over with ease. This is impossible without good information systems and strong linkages between primary and secondary care.

Comment   In all these areas information gives *power*. If putting the patient first is to be more reality than slogan, then much will depend on providing the information for patients to act on. Consider the following questions:

- How can we alter general practitioners' attitudes about encouraging patients to make choices about their care?
- Are practice leaflets not only complete but also comprehensible?
- What issues would patients wish to have addressed in a Patient's Charter for their practice?
- How can the information flow between primary and secondary care be improved?

HEALTH
PROMOTION IN
GENERAL
PRACTICE

A central plank of the government's agenda was highlighted in the title of its White Paper of primary health care: *Promoting Better Health*. General practitioners were considered well-placed to promote good health and prevent ill-health, and their terms of service were altered to include

'giving advice, where appropriate, to a patient in connection with the patient's general health, and in particular about the significance of diet, exercise, the use of tobacco, the consumption of alcohol and the misuse of drugs and solvents' (13(2)(a)).

There were specific requirements in a number of areas which we will consider separately:

- screening and childhood immunization with the introduction of targets;
- children under 5 with the introduction of the Child Health Surveillance List and fee;
- monitoring the health of the adult population through health checks;
- patients over the age of 75 to be offered an annual health check.

The use of targets   Prior to the Contract 'item of service' payments were used to encourage general practitioners to take responsibility in the fields of cervical cytology and childhood immunization. Despite some success in committed practices, these had not succeeded in achieving the required population coverage.

A change in the incentive seemed to be indicated and there was also a desire to shift general practice thinking away from the individual towards the population for which they were responsible. The new approach was remuneration on the basis of achievement of **targets**: to receive payment the general practitioner had to make sure that a target percentage of their eligible patients had undergone the procedure. This meant at least 50% of their women patients had to have a cervical smear, and at least 70% of the children under 5 years had to receive all the appropriate immunizations. There was a higher payment for achieving 80% and 90% respectively. These were initially successful in increasing uptake but a number of issues arose in organization:

- Who was to be included in the at-risk population?
- Were practices or health authorities responsible for the recall procedures?
- How were the staff who carried out the procedures to be trained and supervised?
- Where were the boundaries between informing patients, encouraging them and coercing them to take up procedures?

Failure to address all of these issues led to some confusion and some poorly trained people being involved at first. Despite these difficulties the success of the target approach has led to its extension to other areas of public policy.

Child health   Since before the start of the NHS, Local (Health) Authorities
surveillance   had been responsible for the preventive care of children both before and at school. This included health education and advice,

monitoring growth and development and ensuring immunization uptake. Child welfare clinics and school clinics were run with health visitors and clinic medical officers present.

Some general practitioners became interested in this work, and started to carry out preventive work with under-5's at their own premises. They had a belief that it was important to unite preventive and curative work. This was helped if health visitors were attached to general practices. Some paediatricians and public health doctors were concerned that general practitioners did not have the requisite skills. The discussions went on for many years, but the 1990 Contract encouraged general practitioners to take on this work. In order to do this they have to be eligible for the Child Health Surveillance List, which requires training and experience in the field.

As more general practices take on this work there is less need for local health authority child clinics. As these close down, patients have less choice.

Health checks for adults
For newly registered patients the doctor is expected to enquire about factors of lifestyle which may affect health and to carry out some basic examinations. In the original contract this requirement was extended to all patients who had not been seen for three years.

This move was on much shakier scientific ground than cervical screening or immunization. Doctors were poorly motivated and patient response was poor. In 1993 the approach was changed to a programme of general health promotion to

'improve the health of practice populations by taking action known to be effective on an individual level to reduce morbidity and mortality from coronary heart disease and stroke.'

The new scheme

'sets a framework of national and local priorities ... but allows greater flexibility for practices to develop their own approaches within this' (NHS Management Executive Circular FHSA (93)3).

The framework was a system of three bands (see Box 6.10).

Box 6.10
Health promotion bands

◆ **Band 1:** programmes to reduce smoking.

◆ **Band 2:** programmes to minimize mortality and morbidity of patients at risk from hypertension, or with established coronary heart disease (CHD) or stroke.

◆ **Band 3:** programmes offering a full range of primary prevention of CHD and stroke.

In each band, practices are to collect relevant information on the target population; reach out to people in the priority groups, including those who do not present in the surgery; and offer programmes of intervention which concentrate on lifestyle alteration.

Programmes are to be monitored mainly by reports of the number of patients about whom various factors were recorded, although there is a question about the relationship between recording and intervention.

Despite the comment about 'taking action known to be effective', there is still some concern about the value of these approaches. This concern was fuelled by two large randomized controlled trials of the effectiveness of health checks conducted by nurses in primary care (Imperial Cancer Research Fund OXCHECK Study Group 1994; Family Heart Study Group 1994). Both showed little benefit, although they were intensive programmes and one was designed to use the maximum resources available to general practice.

Keeping an eye on the elderly   A popular innovation was the requirement to offer an annual check for patients over 75, with a home visit if the patient prefers that. This check was to include a review of various aspects of the patient's physical and mental health and well-being, so that appropriate services could be offered.

The debate about health checks for the elderly has continued for many years with little evidence that they are effective in reducing disability or handicap, although more evidence that they improve morale. Harris (1992) has pointed out that part of the problem is knowing what to screen for, and what treatment or advice to offer. It may be more important to find out what people can do than what diseases they are suffering from.

However, a recent study in Holland (Rossum *et al.* 1993) suggested that preventive visits by a nurse looking mainly at function, social contacts, housing and medication did not produce much benefit. As with many authors before, they suggested restricting such visits to subjects in poor health.

Comment   Preventing health problems should, on the whole, make people happier. However, covering a whole population can be expensive and time-consuming. Patients can also get the impression that doctors are more interested in stopping them smoking than in dealing with their anxieties. There is also a danger that doctors become too busy measuring a narrow range of health indicators – such as weight and blood pressure – and this may prevent them thinking out how to approach more urgent needs (such as sexual health and AIDS). GPs will need to consider the questions identified in Box 6.11.

Box 6.11
Questions about health
promotion

♦ What is the best situation for a health promotion initiative: the health centre, the leisure centre, the home or the workplace?

♦ Who are the best people to carry out a health promotion initiative: doctors, practice nurses, public health nurses, health promotion officers or even teachers?

♦ Should GPs be selective with health promotion initiatives: restricting them to people who are known to be in risk groups?

♦ Are GPs flexible in their approaches: can they respond to new needs like promoting sexual health?

THE GENERAL PRACTITIONER AS PURCHASER

The most significant change in the reforms since 1990 has been the development of the role of general practitioners in purchasing. The most obvious element has been the fundholding initiative, but this has led to involvement of general practitioners in district purchasing.

Fundholding

The idea of large practices holding the budget for secondary care was put forward in *Working for Patients* in a fairly tentative way. Various objectives were suggested. Fundholding would:

♦ enable practices to play a more important role in the way NHS money is used to provide services for their patients;
♦ help general practice become a still more satisfying job;
♦ give general practitioners and hospitals a real incentive to put patients first.

The first wave of fundholding in 1991 was small. Within three years it had burgeoned so that a quarter of the population found themselves cared for by GP fundholders. This applied even though only practices (or groups of practices) with a population of over 7000 were considered suitable to hold budgets.

Practices that wanted to be involved in fundholding also had to show that they had the management ability and information systems to do so effectively.

The budget covers six main areas:

♦ a defined group of surgical inpatient and day-case treatment covering most elective procedures;
♦ outpatient services;
♦ diagnostic tests done on an outpatient basis;
♦ drugs and dressings prescribed by the practice;
♦ practice staff;
♦ community health services (only since April 1993).

Even wider trials are being considered (total fundholding is now being widely evaluated). In Hereford and Worcester from 1994 some practices will purchase all kinds of care including emergencies.

The first waves of fundholders had difficulties getting started even though they approached the scheme with enthusiasm and ideas. One study (Glennerster *et al.* 1994) showed how fundholders used their power to promote quality, flexibility and efficiency. Fundholders could also look innovatively at the services they could provide on site – such as purchasing extra outpatient sessions, often practice-based, from consultants, or employing a physiotherapist instead of using drugs for backpain.

Not surprisingly with such a controversial innovation, questions have arisen:

♦ Does fundholding lead to a two-tier service?
♦ Is there a risk that fundholding practices will effectively exclude patients whose care might prove too expensive (cream-skimming)?
♦ Might fixed budgets lead to the danger that some patients who need referral will not get it (under-referral)?

As yet there is no evidence of cream-skimming or under-referral, but fears of a two-tier service have been fuelled by reports of hospitals discontinuing routine operations for the patients of non-fundholders ('because the money in the DHA contract had run out') whilst continuing to admit patients of fundholders.

A number of authors (see Glennerster *et al.* 1994; Roland 1992) have pointed out that some increase in inequality was bound to follow if the scheme was going to be a success, but if fundholding began to address quality issues and improve hospital accountability, this would affect the patients of all doctors.

Purchasing community services has produced its own challenges. Haggard (1993) suggests that savings from other parts of the fund might now be used to purchase additional community services, and thus lead to a redeployment of resources to primary care. But again such purchasing developments increase existing inequalities. Limited community resources (such as trained physiotherapists) need to be shared on the basis of need, equity and effectiveness. Fundholders could upset that, and Haggard perceives that they will have to be involved in choosing between priorities and justifying choices.

Local commissioning Despite its high profile, fundholding is responsible for only a very small amount of the hospital and community budget. It has been calculated that if every person was registered with a fundholder this would still account for only 15% of the budget (Glennerster *et al.* 1994). Most hospital care is still the responsibility of the district health authority as a purchaser. The question was how these purchasers would respond to the challenge of fundholding so that all general practitioners felt the needs of their patients were being considered effectively. Various approaches to commissioning or purchasing at a local level are being tried out. These could be another effective way to ensure that a community's needs are met appropriately in a new more flexible and responsive health service.

Some of these schemes depend on networking local people. Others rely on general practitioners as the advocates of a community's needs (see Wall 1993; Graffy and Williams 1994; Exworthy 1993). General practitioners have been involved by surveys, visits, local forums and through democratic structures such as the **Local Medical Committees (LMCs)**. General practitioners seem to value this involvement and feel their patients could benefit from it; however workload and time constraints prevent many general practitioners, especially in small practices from worrying about purchasing plans.

Fundholders need to be included in this liaison. Much care for their patients is still purchased by the DHA. Fundholders also need to balance their purchasing with the needs of the community. Like non-fundholders they have to work together with community spokespeople and with DHAs (or health commissions) to produce purchasing plans that are geared to the community and not just to an individual practice, even if there is a risk of a circuit back to a planned approach.

General practitioner purchasing The radical innovation of general practitioners as purchasers, whether through fundholding or local commissioning, gives both opportunities and challenges. The opportunities relate to putting pressure on providers to improve the range, accessibility and quality of services and to look at the patients in context. The challenges relate to a number of important questions:

- how to ensure needs are properly assessed (incidentally what is 'need'?);
- how to make available good information about the costs and benefits of available procedures;
- how to promote equity across a range of populations and practices;
- how to balance the patient advocate role with that of a just distributor of limited resources.

The general practitioner in the healthcare marketplace has a number of incentives to improve services generally for the patients of that practice and for the population at large. This means the general practitioner has to learn to manage limited resources. The general practitioner also has a role as an advocate for individual patients, which makes it difficult to distribute resources in a just and equitable way where that means that a particular patient does not get all that money could buy. For instance, patient advocacy may prove a perverse incentive to request an expensive extracontractual referral against general purchasing policy. How general practitioners learn to cope with this tension will be a major factor in the development of primary care in the next decade.

MANAGING AND MONITORING PRIMARY CARE Modern general practice requires many more management skills than it did in 1954. These are required within GP practices, but in the last ten years the FHSAs have also had increased responsibility for planning the organization and development of primary care services.

Practice managers Practice managers are now employed by over three-quarters of practices. There was a steady growth in such appointments over fifteen years but one-fifth of practices made such an appointment in direct response to the increased administrative workload of the 1990 Contract (Greenfield, Nayak and Drury 1991).

Many practice managers work mainly as administrators and bookkeepers. Others have personnel functions relating to non-clinical staff or act as trouble-shooters when there are problems with staff or patients. This can include handling complaints. Fundholding practices also employ fund managers with responsibility for negotiating contracts and other aspects of the budget.

As general practice becomes more complex there are many strategic decisions to be taken about the purposes and priorities of the practice and how these are defined, implemented and monitored through specific policies. This is sometimes carried out by the general practitioners themselves, but in many instances a skilled practice manager can take the lead role in this process.

Managing the contracts General practitioners have always been jealous of their independent contractor status, but demands for a managed and accountable health service have led to an increasing role for the FHSA. To understand how this role may develop in the future it is necessary to consider the changing position of FHSAs and other health authorities.

District health authorities (DHAs) lost responsibility for FHSAs in 1985. Since then their role has changed with the loss of responsibility for direct management of provider services. Both DHAs and FHSAs are involved in purchasing, planning and monitoring of services for broadly similar populations. This has led to closer links in informal and non-statutory health commissions.

As a response to this development, and with a general desire to slim management, the government is introducing enabling legislation to allow statutory merger of the two bodies from 1996. It has stated that the NHS Executive will actively encourage such mergers. Before such mergers take place certain factors need to be considered.

Box 6.12
Some preconditions for a merger of DHAs and FHSAs

◆ *Agreement on populations.* The number of people resident in the district can differ markedly from the number of patients registered with doctors for whom an FHSA is responsible.

◆ *Agreement on contractual arrangements.* DHAs make contracts with provider units, FHSAs have contracts with individual practitioners.

◆ *Agreement on the position of fundholders.* At one level fundholders will be in contract with the purchasing authority; at another level they make their own contracts with provider units which could conflict with purchasing authority priorities.

When these issues are resolved, we can look at the role of the future purchasing authorities in managing primary care. The intended responsibilities have been set out in the government's proposals *Managing the New NHS – A Background Document.* They are:

◆ setting purchasing strategy – targeted to meet local needs;
◆ purchasing services in accordance with local needs;
◆ ensuring delivery of quality and cost targets in contracts;
◆ primary care development;
◆ administration of general practitioners' (and dentists', opticians' and pharmacists') terms of service;
◆ patient registration.

Each raises issues we need to consider in an overview of primary healthcare management. Purchasing services in accordance with local needs has been discussed above, the rest are now considered.

Setting purchasing strategy

Local commissioning requires continuing assessment of local needs. We have seen how purchasers are talking to general practitioners, but such discussions need good information. This should be produced by practices. Annual reports, as required by the 1990 Contract, have been one step towards this. Currently such reports are limited and often subjective. Improvement requires better information systems within practices so that workload activity, referral, hospital usage, and community staff involvement can be monitored effectively.

Prescribing is one aspect of practice activity already monitored in detail through the PACT (Prescribing Analyses and Cost) data. We can look at differences between doctors and discuss factors which might affect prescribing budgets. All non-fundholding doctors are given an 'indicative prescribing budget', and know how much they are expected to spend on pharmaceuticals. Similar information for referrals or investigations is not usually available. Only in a few areas is there effective linkage between hospital and general practice computer systems that would make such analysis easy.

Improved linkage of general practice computer systems with hospitals and FHSAs is a priority, but there is concern about *confidentiality* of clinical data. This needs to be addressed urgently. Capture of anonymous data would provide a picture of local needs that would promote informed approach to strategic planning.

Ensuring delivery to quality and cost targets

Development of appropriate standards and quality targets is a major concern of primary care. People are talking about guidelines for clinical conditions, and about the possibility of individual practice contracts. In some areas of the country Local Medical Committees and FHSAs are coming together to look at standards. They are being assisted by the development of **Medical Audit Advisory Groups** (MAAGs). MAAGs have been one of the major unsung successes of the reforms. Professionally led, they have promoted the debate on standards and quality control in general practice. They have encouraged increasing involvement in audit by both individual practices and by districts. Districts have been able to agree standards for the management of common diseases such as diabetes.

There is a long way to go in developing such standards in the UK although the Dutch College of General Practitioners (NHG) has set a good example (see Box 6.13).

Primary care development

Annual reports have already been mentioned as a contribution to local primary care development. Community care is now a norm for many situations such as mental health and the care of the elderly, previously dealt with in institutions. Community care is the responsibility of local social services departments but it cannot

Box 6.13
The Dutch College of General Practitioners – An example of standard setting

Since 1989 the NHG has published eight or more standards a year, covering areas ranging from acne to varicose veins. Each standard contains:

♦ the NHG standard as published in the Dutch college journal;
♦ a summary (checklist) on a plastic card for day-to-day reference;
♦ a scientific review article, called the scientific justification;
♦ the references;
♦ a teaching package.

Examples have been published in many languages

(Dutch College of General Practitioners (NHG) 1993)

exist without input from primary healthcare teams. We need to work to produce integrated approaches. Some successful experiments are taking place, but general practice will want to know that purchasing authorities are taking a lead in such developments which cannot be dealt with only at a practice level.

Administration of terms of service

FHSAs have been responsible for the administration of centrally agreed contracts and terms of service. In the future contracts might be developed more locally. It has been suggested that purchasing authorities, taking local needs into consideration, should be able to make contracts with individual general practitioners, or (even better) with practices that offer services to fit those local needs. Examples would be a special service for people with drug problems or the homeless, a particular kind of out-of-hours service or cover for a community hospital. Such schemes would need to be careful not to discriminate against a single-handed general practitioner who may not be able to provide the range of services of a large group but does give a much-respected personal service.

Responsibility for contracts also includes investigation of complaints. This will continue but practices are being asked to consider internal complaints procedures so that many incidents can be dealt with early and quickly. There will always be cases when it is not possible to resolve issues at this level. When this happens the grieved parties should be able to turn to a system where the problem can be dealt with quickly and fairly for all concerned. There is currently much concern that procedures are cumbersome and prolonged and can lead to problems of their own.

Patient registration

The last area of responsibility is patient registration. Authorities are responsible for every patient within their area. They have to consider fair and equitable ways of helping those patients who find it difficult to register with a doctor for whatever reason. Some patients are not good at finding a doctor or have difficulties in keeping a good relationship with their doctor. They may be over-demanding, violent and abusive, or they may simply be confused and unable to cope. FHSAs have allocation committees to make sure that patients are registered with a doctor, but they can also assist practices by arranging training in the management of difficult patients.

SUMMARY

This chapter has covered the range of responsibilities of a general practitioner from first contact to the purchase of secondary care when needed.

The responsibility for seeing that every patient has a general practitioner brings us back to the essential principle of primary care services: *All patients must have access to help when they need it.* Management will be concerned with strategies to cope with that demand and to make sure that the limited resources are fairly distributed. Although patients still like to talk about 'my doctor', the doctor is no longer the only person involved in these decisions. The management approach to primary care must therefore take into account various stakeholders in the new situation:

♦ patients;
♦ doctors;
♦ allied health professionals;
♦ practice administrative staff;
♦ government;
♦ purchasers;
♦ providers.

General practices are now considerably stronger in their relationships to secondary care: they provide more and they purchase (or help to commission) more. At the same time they can no longer maintain the same level of total independence that has been traditional. They need to be responsive providers, working under changing contractual arrangements. Even fundholding practices cannot afford to take a totally independent viewpoint. The community-based purchasing system must respond to the total needs of a community, and fundholders must participate in this.

FURTHER READING

♦ Journals: Up-to-date material can be found in *Primary Care Management, British Medical Journal,* and *British Journal of General Practice.*

♦ Marsh, G.N. (1991), *Efficient Care in General Practice*, Oxford University Press, Oxford.

♦ Pritchard, P.M.M. (1984), *Management in General Practice*, Oxford University Press, Oxford.

REFERENCES

Dutch College of General Practitioners (1993), *NHG Standards: 5 Examples of Guidelines for General Practice*. Utrecht: NHG.

Electoral Reform Ballot Services (1992).

Exworthy, M. (1993), The development of purchasing: liaison with GPs, *Primary Care Management*, 3(5):9–10.

Family Heart Study Group (1994), Randomised controlled trial evaluating cardiovascular screening and intervention in general practice: principal results of British family heart study, *BMJ*, 308:313–20.

Glennerster, H., Matsaganis, M., Owen, P. and Hancock, S.P. (1994), Fundholding: wild card or winning hand? In: Robinson, R. and Le Grande, J. (Eds), *Evaluating the NHS Reforms*. Newbury: Policy Journals.

Graffy, J.P. and Williams, J. (1994), Purchasing for all: an alternative to fundholding, *BMJ*, 308:391–4.

Greenfield, S.M., Nayak, A.M. and Drury, M. (1991), *The Impact of*

'Working for Patients' and 'The 1990 Contract' on General Practitioners' Administrative Systems. London: Certified Accountant Publications Ltd.

Haggard, L. (1993), Fundholding and community services, *Primary Care Management*, 3(4):7–8.

Hallam, L. (1993), Access to General Practitioners by telephone: The patient's view. *British Journal of General Practice*, 43:331–5.

Hallam, L. (1994), Primary medical care outside normal working hours: review of published work, *BMJ*, 308:249–53.

Harris, A. (1992), Health checks for people over 75, *BMJ*, 305:599–600.

Imperial Cancer Research Fund OXCHECK Study Group (1994), Effectiveness of health checks conducted by nurses in primary care: results of the OXCHECK study after one year, *BMJ*, 308:308–12.

Mahon, A., Whitehouse, C., Wilkin, D. and Nocon, A. (1993), Factors that influence general practitioners' choice of hospital when referring patients for elective surgery, *British Journal of General Practice*, 43:272–6.

Mahon, A., Wilkin, D. and Whitehouse, C. (1994), Choice of hospital for elective surgery referral: GPs' and patients' views. In: Robinson, R. and Le Grande, J. (Eds), *Evaluating the NHS Reforms*. Newbury: Policy Journals.

Pritchard, P. (1994), The patient's voice in primary health care, *Primary Care Management*, 4(1):6–7.

Rink, E. *et al.* (1993), Impact of introducing near-patient testing for standard investigations in general practice, *BMJ*, 307:775–8.

Roland, M.O. (1992), Fundholding and cash limits in primary care: blight or blessing? In: *The Future of General Practice*. London: British Medical Journal.

Rossum, E.V., Frederiks, C., Philipsen, H. *et al.* (1993), Effects of preventive home visits to elderly people, *BMJ*, 307:27–32.

Sibbald, B., Addington-Hall, J., Brenneman, D. and Freeling, P. (1993), Counsellors in English and Welsh general practices: their nature and distribution. *BMJ*, 306:29–33.

Taylor, S. (1954), *Good General Practice*. London: Oxford University Press.

Wall, A. (1993), Locality purchasing: concept and practice, *Primary Care Management*, 3(7):7–8.

Wiles, R. and Macalister Smith, E. (1993), Counselling in primary care, *Primary Care Management*, 3(8):8–9.

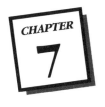

COMMUNITY CARE AND THE HEALTH SERVICE

CHAPTER 7

Martin Knapp and Robyn Lawson

OBJECTIVES

- To show how community care relates to the NHS.

- To describe patterns of need, expenditure, provision, and management of community care.

- To show how government policy and the 1990 Act have influenced the development of community care.

- To identify the key issues which affect the relationship between the NHS and personal social services.

INTRODUCTION

This chapter discusses community care and its relevance for the health service. We begin with a definition, and then describe need, expenditure and service provision. We then outline the development of community care policy, and the major shifts in emphasis introduced by the National Health Service and Community Care Act 1990. We concentrate on some of the issues that are of particular significance at the interface of the NHS and personal social services, and the way in which the recent health and community care reforms seek to tackle them.

The 1990 Act introduced major changes which make it imperative that the health service and local government work closely together. They need to clarify their respective responsibilities and objectives, share their assessment, eligibility and commissioning intentions, and coordinate their complementary commitments to improving the health and welfare of the nation.

There are a number of compelling reasons for closer and compatible working. From a health service perspective, local government responsibilities for community care services are fundamental to the success of the policy aim of reducing inpatient hospital care. The movement towards new service structures for long-term care which received particular emphasis in the 1980s is still not complete, and the deinstitutionalization of long-term care is being followed by increasingly rapid changes in the locus of acute care. Since April 1993, purchasing responsibilities for those residential services which complement deinstitutionalization were transferred from the Department of Social Security to local authority social services departments, making hospital discharges to long-stay care dependent on local authority assessments of need. Other less obvious examples of the interdependence between the two statutory agencies include the importance of local government housing, education, road building and leisure services to the attainment of health gain targets.

WHAT IS COMMUNITY CARE?   Community care is associated with a particular set of user or client groups (sometimes within the health service referred to as **'priority care groups'**). Numerically, the largest user groups are elderly people, and people with physical and learning disabilities, mental health problems, addiction or substance abuse problems, HIV/AIDS or sensory impairments. Care of children in need of support or substitute family provision tends to be discussed separately, and is governed by a different set of legislative instruments. We follow precedent and largely exclude discussion of child care services from this chapter, though this is not to deny the importance of close collaboration between child health and social services.

The term 'community care' has been used to mean a number of different things, which has generated inevitable difficulties of interpretation and communication. Community care, as the term is now used in government policy, incorporates a number of elements (see Box 7.1).

These are the principal elements of community care identified in *Caring for People* the White Paper which preceded the radical changes introduced by the 1990 Act.

Box 7.1
Key elements of community care

- It refers to the policy of enabling people to live as normal a life as possible in their own homes or in domestically-scaled environments in the community.

- It generally means aiming to provide the right amount of care and support to help people achieve maximum possible independence and, by acquiring or re-acquiring basic living skills, to help them to achieve their full potential.

- It implies giving people greater influence over how they live their lives and the services they need to help them to do so.

Box 7.2
The ageing of the
population

Between 1951 and 1987 the number of people in the UK aged over 65 rose from 5.5 million to 8.8 million. This age group now comprises 15% of the total population, compared to 11% in 1951. Projections indicate that the proportion of older people in the population will remain fairly constant over the next decade, but that there will be a substantial increase in the early part of the next century as the post-war 'baby boom' group reaches retirement age. Although the overall number of elderly people will show a slight decline in the next decade, there will be a significant ageing of elderly people. It is projected there will be a rise of 600 000 people over the age of 75 between the late 1980s and 2001, while the number of people aged 85 years and over will increase by 75% over the same period to comprise 13% of all older people (Harrison and Means 1990).

THE SCALE OF NEED FOR COMMUNITY SERVICES

The ageing of the population (see Box 7.2) is often seen as problematic by policymakers and politicians because of the higher incidence of illness and disability in old age, and the associated needs for health and social care, together with changing needs for housing, pensions and income maintenance, assistance with transport and so on. An ageing population also means that while more people as a proportion of the total are dependent on services provided by the welfare system, fewer people are paying for that system through national insurance contributions and general taxation, putting pressure on the Exchequer and the welfare state in general.

An OPCS study of the prevalence of physical and learning disabilities in the UK in the mid 1980s showed that five adults per thousand of the population are in the highest severity category for disability used in that particular survey, and, overall, 142 adults per thousand have some type or degree of disability.

It is important to emphasize that estimates of the overall prevalence of disability depend on the concepts and methods used, so that estimates produced by different studies may bear no direct relationship to each other, although they may indicate similar trends. However, it is clear that disability is more common among older groups of people and that a majority of the most severely disabled are living in communal establishments (Martin *et al*. 1988). Altogether there are 1.3 million people in England who are registered disabled, 6% of whom have very severe disabilities (Department of Health 1992).

The overall prevalence of severe learning disability (sometimes referred to as 'mental handicap') in the UK is usually estimated as being in the order of three or four people per thousand population. However, different mortality rates mean that, as the population ages, the proportion with the greatest level of learning disability falls. A recent register-based study in North West Thames Region suggested that the rate is 3.7–3.8 per 1000 among the population aged 15–44; among 45–64 years old a 'true' prevalence rate of 2.4 per 1000 is projected; and 1.25 per 1000 in the population aged over 65 (Farmer *et al.* 1991).

With regard to community mental health services, where local authority housing and social services departments are becoming increasingly involved as providers or purchasers in an area previously dominated by the health service, estimating incidence and prevalence is fraught with difficulties owing to the lack of consensus over definitions and diagnoses. The relative responsibilities of the two public authorities, and of non-statutory agencies, vary between diagnostic groups. For example, it is estimated that the incidence of schizophrenia is three or four adults in every thousand, with a typical district health authority with a population of 250 000 expecting between 20 and 40 new cases each year. But the cost contribution of local authorities prior to the 1993 implementation of the funding route changes for residential care and nursing homes was estimated to be only 6% of total cost (Kavanagh *et al.* 1993a). In contrast, local authorities accounted for 23% of the expenditure on support for the estimated 541 000 elderly people with dementia in England (Kavanagh *et al.* 1993b).

THE SCALE OF EXISTING PROVISION

Since the 1990 Act came into force, local authorities have had lead responsibility for community social care, with statutory obligations to work closely with certain other agencies for some activities. As we illustrate below, links with the health service are not always straightforward. The statutory powers and obligations of social services departments include the provision (or commissioning) of:

> services for vulnerable children and families, elderly people with social difficulties, mentally ill, mentally handicapped, physically ill, sensorally impaired and physically disabled people and the homeless. (House of Commons Health Committee 1991, HC409-i, 43)

Expenditure and funding

Local authority services or purchases are funded by a number of sources. The three main sources have traditionally been:

- local taxes (formerly the rates and Community Charge or poll tax, and now the Council Tax);
- the unhypothecated general revenue support grant from central government (allocated on the basis of a negotiated formula which in part reflects differences in needs and costs) and
- user charges for services (which have declined in relative importance to around 10% of the total).

There are also a number of specific grants from central government, some of which are targeted on particular user groups – for instance the **Mental Illness Specific Grant**, and grants for social care support for people with HIV/AIDS. In addition there are relatively small amounts of money which have been set aside to encourage collaborative service development. These include joint finance and 'dowry' payments which are made by health authorities under Section 28A of the NHS Act 1977 to local authorities, housing associations and voluntary organizations to pay for personal social services, education for disabled people, and housing.

Overall spending on the personal social services has grown since Mrs Thatcher became Prime Minister: Wistow and Manning (1993) calculate that inflation-adjusted expenditure was 40.6% greater in 1992/93 than in 1978/79, equivalent to an annual rate of 2.9%. This is a lower rate of growth than that claimed by the government, the difference being due to Wistow and Manning's use of the specific social services inflation index to weight spending. Nevertheless, even this lower growth measure is in excess of the figure of 2% historically agreed by government and the local authorities to be necessary to keep pace with demographic and other needs-related pressures.

In 1992/93, the year before the final phase of implementation of the 1990 Act, net current expenditure on the personal social services in England was £5 billion. In April 1993, an additional £565 million was transferred to English local authorities from the Department of Social Security in the form of the **Special Transitional Grant** (STG). This major new source of local authority social services funding moves money over a four-year period from the social security vote to local authority social care (eventually amounting to a sum which will be almost a third of total social care expenditure in 1992). Prior to the introduction of the STG, the general revenue support grant from central government represented about 80% of total local authority income, having grown appreciably in size during the 1990s (Knapp and Wistow 1993b). From 1997/98 funding for community care will no longer be separately identified, however, but will be channelled through the revenue support grant once more, and distributed between authorities in the normal way on the basis of their standard spending assessments.

Recently published statistics from the Department of Health disaggregate local authority expenditure by user groups (see Box 7.3). It can be seen that two user groups (elderly people and children) account for more than three-quarters of all spending on the personal social services. There have been few changes over the 12-year period, though the larger amount allocated to the support of people with learning disabilities, physical disabilities and mental health problems is indicative, in part, of the changing balance of

Box 7.3
Personal social
services net
percentage
expenditure by client
groups

Client group	1978/79	1990/91
Elderly	45.4	44.2
Children	37.4	34.4
Learning disabilities	9.6	13.1
Physical disabilities	4.8	5.0
Mental health problems	1.9	2.4
Other	0.9	0.9

Source: Department of Health, OPCS and HM Treasury (1993), *Department of Health and Office of Population Censuses and Surveys, Departmental Report*, Cm 2212, London HMSO.

responsibilities between health and social care, and particularly the trend away from long-stay hospital accommodation for these user groups in favour of community-based support.

Service provision   There are four main service provider sectors – informal, statutory, voluntary, and private for-profit.

Easily the largest is the *informal care sector*, principally comprising individual carers (family members and others). As we describe below, the 1990 Act laid particular emphasis on the need for local and health authorities to 'care for the carers' – to provide support and respite services and coordination through care or case management, and to involve them in decision-making.

We have already described the main *public sector* agency – the local authority social services department – in terms of its patterns of expenditure and sources of income, but other local government services (such as education and housing) have important roles to play, as obviously do hospitals, community and primary healthcare services. Furthermore the Department of Social Security remains a major source of funding for many people through the benefit system.

The independent sector is also, and increasingly, an important source of provision. The *voluntary sector* is comprised of organizations which are independent of government and, although they may earn profits, are bound by the 'non-distribution constraint', which means that they cannot distribute the profits to any owners or shareholders. Many voluntary organizations have charitable status, conferring certain tax advantages.

The *private sector* is also constitutionally separate from government, but aims to be profit-earning and profit-distributing. In recent years, the private sector has become a very much more important provider of social services, especially of residential care and nursing home services.

The chief types of services provision are domiciliary, day and residential care.

Domiciliary care

The home help service, provided mainly by local authority social services departments (although independent sector provision is growing slowly), plays an important role in enabling people to remain living in their own homes and in supporting carers. There are no recent figures for provision, but as the population ages and demand grows, local authorities, spurred on by central government (see, for example, Social Services Inspectorate 1987), are increasingly trying to target services on the most dependent people. The most common domiciliary service provided by local authorities is the meals service. More than 45 million meals were delivered in 1991/92, three-quarters of them in people's own homes (Social Services Inspectorate 1993).

Day care

Day care provision has increased over the past ten years, although in parts of the country and for certain user groups there remain shortages. For example, there was a 50% increase in the number of local authority day centres between 1981 and 1991, so that there are now more than 1500 centres with 60 100 places. Provision in adult training centres and special needs units for people with learning disabilities grew by 30% over the same period (Social Services Inspectorate 1993).

Residential care

There were 288 600 adults in (staffed) residential accommodation in March 1992. The majority (83%) were described in Department of Health statistics as 'elderly people', another 10% were people with learning disabilities, 3% had mental health problems and 3% had physical disabilities. The other 1% included drug and alcohol misusers.

The numbers of people in residential care grew by an enormous amount over the 1980s. For example, the number of places in homes for elderly and younger physically disabled people increased by 57% between 1980 and 1991, with the private sector growing by more than 300%. The private sector's market share leapt from 19% to 54% and it had displaced the public sector as the largest provider by 1988. There were similar, if less marked trends in the inter-sectoral balance of provision in relation to residential services for people with learning disabilities and mental health problems (Wistow *et al.* 1994).

Comment

The nature of community care is changing quite rapidly as providers in all sectors, but especially private and voluntary organizations, develop new and innovative services, and as users and carers increasingly come to impose their preferences on provider responses. This means that the generic labels for services used above – 'day care' and 'residential care' – now refer to a very wide variety of service types and inherent objectives. It also means that some of the new facilities and arrangements now being introduced do not fit comfortably, if at all, within these categories.

Unintended consequences

The huge expansion of the private residential and nursing home sectors was the biggest change in community care in the 1980s and early 1990s. It is widely interpreted as an unintended consequence of what was said by the government at the time to be simply clarification and subsequently equalization of social security funding entitlements, which made it possible for elderly and other adults to obtain ready access to non-statutory homes without assessment of their care needs.

Government Miscalculation

The combined effect of this liberal social security regime and the fiscal constraints on local government can be seen in relation to market shares in the largest of the residential care sectors – supporting elderly people and younger adults with physical disabilities (Figure 7.1).

Many people who could probably have managed well in the community with a modest amount of home care support found the financial advantages and relative security of publicly funded residential care to be very attractive. By March 1991, 60% of elderly people in private and voluntary sector residential care in England

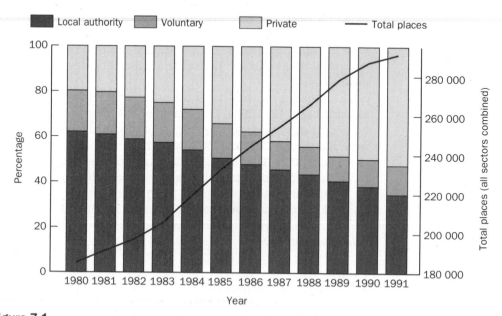

Figure 7.1
Percentage by sector and total residential places for elderly and younger physically handicapped people

Sector and principal funding source and client group	Percentages of residents in each sector's old people's homes funded from different sources				
	Inner London	*Outer London*	*Metropolitan districts*	*Shire counties*	*All authorities*
Local authority homes					
Local authority funding[1]	100	100	100	100	100
Private and voluntary homes					
Income support[2]	66.2	59.0	71.5	56.8	59.7
Local authority contracts[2]	25.3	8.4	1.0	0.5	1.6
Private means and other sources[3]	8.5	32.7	27.5	42.6	38.7

[1] 27% of local authority spending on these homes is covered by fees and charges to residents.
[2] Includes top-ups by residents, families or homes.
[3] Privately funded or funded from organizations' own income (charitable donations, investments).

Box 7.4
Sources of funding for residents of old people's homes, England, March 1991

were funded by the DSS via income support (many of them further subsidized from other sources, including the homes themselves), compared with 14% in 1979 and 36% in the mid-1980s (House of Commons Social Services Committee 1985; Ernst and Whinney 1986). Another 2% were funded by local authorities, and the remaining 39% funded themselves or (if they were in voluntary sector homes) may have been supported in part or in whole by charitable donations or organizations' other income sources (see Box 7.4). Income support payments for care in private and voluntary residential and nursing homes totalled £1300 million in March 1991, and perhaps as much as £2480 million by April 1993, compared with supplementary benefit payments of £10 million in 1979 (Henwood *et al.* 1991; Hansard 1993).

The growth in the demand for independent sector residential and nursing home care during the 1980s was met with a mixed **supply-side** response. As noted above, the private sector responded most rapidly and successfully. The costs of setting up a home were relatively low: for example, in many areas of the country there was a low-priced supply of suitable premises (small guesthouses and former hotels), and banks and other financial institutions were very willing to make loans. Future prospects looked excellent, and the private sector was able easily to raise the equity capital necessary to finance new ventures. However, the huge and, for the government, expensive increase in supply was a key reason for subsequent policy developments aimed at curbing future growth.

This seller's market has been changed overnight into a much less rosy prospect for those individuals and companies who have sunk large sums into their businesses. Since local authority social services departments assumed responsibility for funding residential care in April 1993, fewer people are being placed in these homes than had previously referred themselves with the support of social security payments. Moreover, some local authorities are driving hard bargains on price and quality of care.

THE DEVELOPMENT OF COMMUNITY CARE POLICY

The beginnings of community care as a concept can be traced back to the 1920s, but the term came to prominence more generally in the early 1970s with the beginnings of the movement to rehabilitate long-stay patients in the community. Even then the term 'community care' was the subject of some confusion as to whether it was a description of the services or resources involved (for example, those services provided outside of institutions), or a statement of objectives.

Until recently, the role of government in community care policy has looked more reactive than proactive. As Goodwin commented, the introduction of a community care policy by the Ministry of Health in the 1950s was 'not so much generating a new and progressive policy as responding to changing circumstances' (1989, p. 45). It followed rather than shaped professional opinion and preferences, and was undoubtedly encouraged and buffeted by economic forces. For example, the reforms contained within the 1959 Mental Health Act, like earlier government statements, sought to foster or establish not community care for people with mental health problems, but 'treatment in the community'. These reforms were necessary to overcome problems already arising as a result of changes in professional practice and political–economic theories 'Rather than simply constituting a reformist measure resulting from enlightened thinking, the community care policy in fact represented a response to a crisis of institutional care' (Goodwin 1989, p. 41).

A similar trend can be seen if we look at hospital rundown policies of the past 40 years. The 1975 White Paper, *Better Services for the Mentally Ill* (Cmnd 6233), posited that community care would be cheaper than hospital, though the DHSS's 1981 consultative document was more circumspect, and subsequent statements have generally shied away from any assumption of *major* cost benefits from hospital closure. These views from central government were based upon fairly comprehensive cost concepts. A more partial or fragmented view of costs, such as a health authority calculating only its own expenditure implication of hospital closure, would likely encourage over-enthusiastic support for such a policy, and introduces the danger of the under-funding of community care (Knapp 1994).

In spite of the difficulties encountered in making community care a reality, there has never been a time when it has been more important, both to government and to the service users and their families who stand to benefit, that such a policy should succeed. Growing awareness of demographic trends, coupled with social trends reducing the number of available carers, have served to heighten concern about the future costs and availability of care. Together with **macroeconomic** difficulties in the last two decades, and the huge growth in expenditure on residential and nursing home care, there are powerful incentives for the government to control expenditure, but growing concomitant needs for more or better support.

Because policy and practice have developed in an expedient rather than rational way, there is no clear definition of what community care is or what it can achieve. Bulmer (1987) identified four different usages of the term.

♦ Its original meaning was care outside of large institutions, meaning anything other than the remote and massive asylums, erected during the Victorian era to keep the 'feeble minded' (as they were called) apart from the general public, for their assumed mutual benefit.

♦ A second meaning was the delivery of various professional services outside of all hospitals, as in 'community nursing' or 'community mental health terms'.

♦ Thirdly, it could connote care *by* the community, principally via the involvement of voluntary agencies and families. The inequity of the informal care burden was addressed, though not necessarily resolved, by the 1990 Act.

♦ Finally, community care has been used to describe provision which is as close to normality or ordinary living as possible.

These definitions are still in use, and elements of each of them are embodied in the government's view of community care described earlier. Consequently there have been differences in, and difficulties of, interpretation and communication. From a health service perspective, for instance, community care was seen for many years simply as getting people out of hospital. Quite what was to happen thereafter was not tackled thoroughly in official publications. The 1971 White Paper on mental handicap services, for instance, included rather unspecific strategies for the support of service users and families, and only one of the five main policy objectives made recommendations for services in the community (Wistow 1985).

For many years, therefore, community care was encouraged as a 'Good Thing'. But it was not supported via any particular financial incentives until the arrival of joint finance in the 1970s, and was then fettered by so many disincentives and limitations as to lead the House of Commons Social Services Committee (1985, para 21) to complain of 'underfinanced and understaffed' community provision. The ready access to residential care funded by the DSS provided an additional disincentive to invest in community services. Walker described the history of community care as 'painfully slow progress towards timid goals' (1982, p. 16), and the House of Commons Social Services Committee (1985) complained that 'community care [had] become a slogan, with all the weakness that implies' (para 8); it was not a rounded policy.

There is a strong case for arguing that a community care policy *per se* that is a policy in which community care was the primary and not the residual aim did not arrive until the late 1980s. The highly critical report from the Audit Commission, *Making a Reality of Community Care* (1986), highlighted the anomalies and organizational inefficiencies of a system dominated by perverse incentives, poor targeting and wasted resources. The outcomes of the system included:

♦ the enormous drain on social security revenue represented by access to residential and nursing home care without adequate assessment of care needs;
♦ the uncompensated, inequitable burdens placed on family carers, especially women;
♦ the slow rate of development of community facilities in relation to the speed of hospital rundown;
♦ the lack of community-based alternatives to residential care; and
♦ the neglect of disabled people without adequate assistance, supervision or personal resources.

This Audit Commission report was highly influential in the government's commissioning of Sir Roy Griffiths' review of community care (1988), on which were based the White Paper, *Caring for People*, and the 1990 National Health Services and Community Care Act.

THE COMMUNITY CARE REFORMS The 1989 White Paper addressed the various and increasingly damaging weaknesses of the community care system. These weaknesses or problems had contributed to the slow, uneven and misshapen development of community services. The speed with which the 1989 *NHS and Community Care Bill* followed the White Paper (nine months between publication of one and Enactment of the other) is indicative of the importance which the government attached to these (and the health service) reforms.

The Act introduced the most sweeping changes to health and social welfare services seen in the UK since the 1940s. These reforms to community social care can be summarized as the encouragement of movement along four core strategic dimensions. (This dimensionality and some of the ideas which flow from it were developed by Martin Knapp and Gerald Wistow in work with the Social Services Inspectorate (1992).)

The balance between institutional and community care

The 1990 Act – and central government policy more generally – explicitly encourage local authorities to shift the emphasis away from institutional in favour of domiciliary-based care, just as there is 'strategic shift' between acute and community care in the health service. Thus the separation of purchasers from providers in health has been combined with rapid developments in community-based clinical procedures dramatically to reduce the utilization of hospital inpatient services. There are equivalent changes in community social care.

The combination of changes to the funding and commissioning routes and growing experience with community-based organization and delivery of care (especially through care or case management) are shifting the balance in social care. There are now far stronger incentives for local authorities to substitute domiciliary-based care for more expensive residential and nursing home services. Long-term hospital provision is also being run down in favour of (it is hoped) well-supported care in the community, and the use of residential and nursing home care is being discouraged when good-quality support can be provided in domiciliary settings.

Supply-led versus needs-led care

The second strategic objective of central government policy which can be readily distinguished in a number of specific actions is to move the community care system away from supply-led, provider-dominated services – a general feature of post-war social policy across almost all areas, from education and housing to health and welfare – to a system of needs-led, purchaser-dominated services.

In the new environment of the 1990s, it is intended that services be much more sensitive and responsive to the needs and preferences of users and their carers. User and carer representatives are being added to planning and other groups. Care or case management is strongly encouraged by the Department of Health to assess needs and identify the preferences of users and carers, and then to coordinate the service responses. In some local authorities, such as in Kent, care managers (individuals or teams) hold devolved budgets (actual or shadow) with which to purchase services from a range of providers.

Increased pluralism

The third core dimension of the 1990 Act is the explicit, indeed heavy, emphasis on the mixed economy of care. Specifically, this means the encouragement of greater **pluralism** in provision with markedly greater roles for private and voluntary agencies.

Some local authorities have responded by creating new, hybrid 'not-for-profit' agencies, often built around floated-off local authority services. There are new forms of regulation of provision through contractual as well as grant-aid links and through quality assurance. In the longer term, though this remains no more than a controversial gleam in the ministerial eye, there may need to be greater variety of funding sources. The last of these is certainly not current government policy, but broad public policy debate of private long-term care insurance is going to be inevitable very soon, and insurance companies are busily researching the market.

Divergent demographic and economic trends described earlier will force radical thoughts and will need imaginative action. In this respect, of course, the community care reforms share a number of features with the longer term and broader privatization thrust of the Thatcher and Major governments.

The balance between NHS and local funding

The final element of government community care policy, though one which initially received less attention than the others, is alteration of the balance of responsibility for decision-making and funding between the National Health Service and local government. This has mainly been achieved through the transfer of funds from the Department of Social Security to social services departments, and the latter being given the lead role in community care. The intention is to improve collaboration and coordination in planning, commissioning and the provision of services.

One of the reasons why the problems of formulating and implementing a successful community care policy remained intractable for so long was that the services which make community care possible are many and various. They include day care and day hospital, home helps and community nurses, meals on wheels, and supported housing (such as sheltered housing and group homes). Acute care and long-stay care in residential and nursing homes are also needed as back-ups to care provided in domiciliary settings. Responsibility for provision of these services spans a number of agencies, and the distinction between health and social care has not always been clear-cut. Housing departments (which are separate from social services departments in county council areas) also have a fundamental part to play. The resultant confusion and occasional friction between agencies have meant both yawning gaps and wasteful overlaps in provision.

THE NHS/LA INTERFACE It is an explicit government hope that changes flowing from the NHS and Community Care Act 1990 will make inter-agency collaboration easier to achieve between health and local authorities, and also between the statutory and non-statutory sectors. By shifting substantial additional purchasing power to local authorities and giving them the lead role in community care, stronger incentives have been created for closer and more productive working between the various players. For instance, health authorities – if they do not wish to pay for the placements themselves, and if users cannot afford them – cannot now discharge hospital inpatients to nursing or residential homes without the agreement of local authority social services departments.

Nevertheless, following implementation of the 1990 Act there are now more agencies and other players in the mixed economy than before. The new constellation of health and social care agencies and the main funding connections between them are represented diagrammatically in Figure 7.2. This diagram is not complete – it ignores some of the small or emerging financial connections (such as joint commissioning) – but still amply illustrates two key points.

♦ First, a complex network of vertical and horizontal relationships must be negotiated if individuals in need are to be provided with

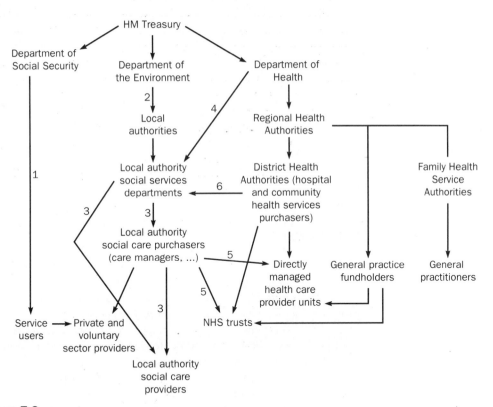

Figure 7.2

Finding routes in health and social care in England in 1992 (source: Knapp and Wistow 1993a)

1. Social security funding via individual claimants
2. Annual Revenue Support Grant
3. Purchaser–provider split is not operated across all local authorities
4. Special Transitional Grant and other specific grants (mental health, drugs and alcohol, ...)
5. Only when trusts or DMUs provide social care
6. Joint finance and Section 28A payments

integrated, continuous and perhaps 'seamless' care (Wistow 1991, 1992; Knapp and Wistow 1993a).
♦ Second, top-down policy initiatives from government can still, generally, only take the form of advice and encouragement, not binding directives. Incentives need to be in place.

There remains the danger, therefore, that the reforms will produce organizational fragmentation and confusion, with little improvement on the features identified by the Audit Commission as characteristic of the system in the 1980s.

Better coordination of these services at the macro level might be achieved via closer and better links between the main statutory and independent agencies involved in provision and purchasing, and at the micro level through the appropriate and clearer delegation of 'case' or 'patch' responsibilities and the involvement in key decisions of individual service users and their families. The DoH guidance which followed the 1990 Act explicitly encouraged both macro and micro coordination, with jointly developed annual **Community Care Plans**, joint commissioning, and 'bottom-up' care management. Most of these feature carer and user involvement in decision-making. The process and potential of each of these is discussed below.

(margin handwritten note: POSSIBLE SOLUTION)

COMMUNITY CARE PLANNING

Caring for People reintroduced formal requirement for social services departments to plan services locally, but in a different way from the old norm- and guideline-based planning of the 1970s. The new form of planning is consistent with new forms of management; it is oriented towards mapping, managing and monitoring markets, and should be less bureaucratic and centralized than earlier arrangements. For instance, the emphasis of collaboration is on the achievement of agreed priorities and outcomes rather than on process. By giving local authority social services departments the central planning role to assess and meet need and to ration services by assessment, *Caring for People* stopped short of committing the personal social services to full 'marketization'. The market is not allowed to allocate resources between users – providers must compete, but users will not (Kelly 1991). Furthermore, there is a more explicit link between population needs assessment and resource allocation, in that resources are allocated to some extent on the basis of assessed need (as laid out in community care plans), at least until 1997/98 when community care resources from central government will no longer be separately identified.

Each social services department must build up a population profile identifying need and available supply, and produce three-year community care plans which are updated annually. These plans must be produced in consultation with users, carers and the independent sector, and collaboratively with local DHAs, FHSAs and housing authorities. However, as Wistow, Leedham and Hardy (1993) found from their detailed examination of 25 of the first community care plans (prepared for 1992/93), it was by no means common for all parties to be equal stakeholders or even apparently represented.

With the more complex organizational and funding environment introduced by the reforms, *computerized management and financial information systems* have become yet more important, and ought to play a vital role in linking needs identified at the individual 'case' level with the population needs assessment which is an integral part of the community care planning process. In the absence of information systems, two of the key aims of the 1990 reforms – devolution of decision-making and of financial responsibility (for example, for purchasing) – will be much more difficult to achieve. For this reason, many local authorities are delaying the devolution of powers until they have fully operational information systems.

Even so, most local authorities recognize that the information which they input to their new systems is itself in need of development. For example, cost and outcome indicators remain poor. FHSAs have a major role to play in ensuring that the views of GPs, including fundholders, and primary healthcare teams, are properly reflected in discussions and negotiations with social services departments. They should be active participants in the development of community care plans. This ability to plan primary care is relatively new and widely welcomed, though there is relatively little evidence yet of major beneficial effects on community care. In addition, FHSAs can apply incentives for GPs to undertake certain types of work; they can tap into GP knowledge of local communities; and they can represent GPs in collaborative work with health and local authorities. Furthermore, the computerized patient registers being developed by GPs have the potential to provide valuable information for planning purposes.

As purchasers, GP fundholders have a particular interest in community care plans, for instance in the overall strategy and principles which health and social services agree for purchasing community care, including any assumptions about the balances between residential and nursing home care, day and domiciliary provision, respite services, and so on. DoH guidance urges fundholders to share their purchasing intentions with DHAs and other fundholders, so that DHAs, which are the main link to social services departments, can feed this information into the community care planning process (EL(92)48).

Joint commissioning   Commissioning can be interpreted broadly to comprise a number of linked tasks. These run from agreement of a mission statement through assessment, service specification and contracting, to information feedback. Taken together, these activities imply both a shift from an administrative to a management culture, and a strengthening of those planning and purchasing activities which, historically, have been underdeveloped.

Wertheimer and Greig (1993) have usefully characterized **joint commissioning** as comprising a number of features (a mixture of tasks and desirable attributes), building on the work of Knapp and Wistow (1993a). These are listed in Box 7.5.

Box 7.5
Features of joint commissioning

◆ 'Money in the same pot', though not necessarily shared or merged financial systems.

◆ Joint decisions about how that money is spent.

◆ A shared set of values in a climate of mutual trust.

◆ Joint commissioning as a means to improve outcomes for users and carers.

◆ A commitment to improved quality in services.

◆ An aim to achieve coherence at all levels of commissioning and purchasing, from macro commissioning to micro purchasing.

◆ Recognition that there will be gains and losses, and compromises to authority and autonomous decision-making powers, though not to their values.

◆ Individual organizations retain the ability to discharge their statutory responsibilities in ways which enable them to retain accountability.

Some commissioning tasks occur at a macro (or strategic) level, some at a micro (or tactical) level, and some at both levels. *Macro-level commissioning* is the responsibility of whole authorities, or large parts thereof, and can be conducted either singly or jointly by health and local authorities. It includes population needs assessments and the production of community care plans as described earlier, and is often characterized by centralized budgets and large block contracts. By contrast, *micro-level commissioning* is the responsibility of individual care managers or teams. It involves individual needs assessments, the tailoring of authority plans to local circumstances and individual potentialities, for example in relation to devolved budgets and spot purchasing (Knapp & Wistow 1993b).

Joint commissioning involves some pooling of resources, and clarity about aims and methods. The opportunities for joint commissioning are thus more likely to arise when

♦ there is an overlapping responsibility or domain of activity;
♦ when health and local authorities are dependent on a common (external) resource pool; and/or
♦ when one agency is heavily dependent on the other for funding or needs bombardment.

Two of the service areas which have seen the development of joint commissioning initiatives are *discharge planning* (from hospital) and *care for people with learning disabilities* (Henwood and Wistow 1993; Wertheimer and Greig 1993). Macro-level joint commissioning is developing slowly but significantly, while at a micro-level there may also be opportunities for joint purchasing, with care managers pooling resources with fundholding GPs, or operating from a single site to facilitate the joint micro-commissioning and monitoring roles in general. Indeed the creation of joint structures (such as joint commissioning agencies) and the pooling of resources are important means to, and products of, successful collaboration more broadly defined.

The benefits of joint commissioning are that it offers, for example, the opportunity for greater flexibility and coordination across agencies. There is the more effective use of available resources, reducing the likelihood of overlaps and gaps in service responses. It therefore provides the chance to settle the old dispute about what are nursing tasks and what are home care tasks. This should mean the potential for better targeting of resources on needs. From a procedural standpoint, joint commissioning improves the prospects of moving to clearer and more consistent eligibility criteria. It should raise mutual awareness, foster cooperation rather than competition, and weaken previous tendencies to shunt people and costs on to other agencies. For example, joint commissioning of residential and nursing home care increases the likelihood of achieving a more appropriate balance between congregate and community care across the health and social care system as a whole.

Care management Care or case management, where micro-commissioning takes place, is one of the central planks of government community care policy. Care management arrangements in Britain have been explored most extensively in the coordination of services for elderly people (Challis and Davies 1986; Davies and Challis 1986; Challis *et al.* 1988, 1990). The results of these experiments encouraged both the Audit Commission (1986) and Sir Roy Griffiths (1988) to advocate care management as a key component of community care reforms.

Care management is 'the lynch-pin of an individual needs-led service' (Audit Commission 1989, para 49), the 'glue that binds otherwise fragmented services into arrangements that respond to the unique and changing needs' of clients (Freedman and Moran

Box 7.6
Five core tasks of care
management

- ◆ Case finding and referral.
- ◆ Assessment and selection.
- ◆ Care planning and service packaging.
- ◆ Monitoring and reassessment.
- ◆ Case closure.

1984, p. 23). The process comprises five core tasks as listed in Box 7.6 (Davies and Challis 1986):

Underpinning care management, and particularly the case planning and monitoring tasks, is some form of individual programme, service or care planning. To the politician, care management offers the opportunity to mix the economy of social care without reorganizing agencies, whilst to the user or carer it should mean a single access point and support for participation, representation and choice. Care management is argued to be one way to improve the efficiency and equity of resource allocation, although the many parties to community care policy and practice decisions may not agree what or whose efficiency or equity should have priority.

Care management may take place in hospital or community settings, and may not all be undertaken by the same person or team, especially where joint assessments and care planning by social services and health practitioners are required for someone with complex needs. Problems have been encountered in designing ways of conducting joint assessments – for instance in designing an assessment tool which is relevant and usable by the different actors involved.

GPs have a role to play in needs-based assessment and service access for individual people, and FHSAs will have a key role in keeping GPs and primary healthcare teams informed of developments and in ensuring that their views are reflected as far as possible in agreements reached with social services departments. Fundholding general practices will have an impact in relation to micro-commissioning, and will need to know about the criteria for eligibility for different levels of health and social care (including nursing home and residential care) which are agreed between health and social services and which will feed into the assessment process (EL(92)48). However, there is as yet no real health care equivalent to the care management role within community care.

PARTICULAR   Commissioners and providers face a number of both general and
CHALLENGES   specific challenges in relation to those needs and services which

reside in the so-called grey area between health and social services, where provision could come from both or neither public agency, where guidance on responsibility is often complex, and where the case for a joint or coordinated approach is consequently strong. These grey areas often lie at another interface also: that between primary, acute and long-stay care. Examples include hospital discharge schemes, the provision of continence advice treatment and products, respite care, and reprovision of long-stay hospitals (see Lawson 1993, for details).

'Home from hospital'

'Home from hospital' and 'home from hospice' schemes provide intensive rehabilitation or hospice-type service in people's own homes to facilitate discharge from acute hospital beds. It is believed that these services not only help patients to recover faster, but also that they can prevent readmission and longer term dependence on, for instance, community nurses and home helps. 'Home from hospital' care can therefore represent an efficient use of resources, with clear benefits for users, and health and local authorities alike. 'Home from hospital' services bridge the gap between hospital care and community care, and can be managed by the health authority, local authority, or a voluntary organization on their behalf. For instance, there are schemes operated by district nurses, local authority home helps and Age Concern groups.

Since such schemes rely on good liaison and cooperation between staff of different agencies, there is scope to create joint schemes. In Bexley, Kent, for example, arrangements are being piloted to bring the health authority's community nursing service and the local authority's home help service into joint operation in teams centred on GP practices. This will enable the planning and delivery of care to be undertaken in ways which are more flexible, responsive and creative than can usually be achieved under the traditional, separate arrangements. This may eventually lead to a jointly commissioned service. 'Home from hospital' schemes are being piloted within this context, funded using joint finance and local authority funding to the voluntary sector (Lawson 1993).

Continence services

Another grey area between health and local authority responsibility is provision of a continence service. Incontinence can precipitate the breakdown of informal care arrangements and lead to admission to long-term care. However, the purchase of continence advice and products which can help prevent or manage incontinence is often confused by unclear responsibilities for health and local authorities, especially in relation to provision for people in residential and nursing homes. It is not uncommon for both agencies to be looking to limit or even reduce their expenditure in this field. Furthermore, the creation of trusts in the NHS means that continence advisers may be employed either by an acute trust or a community trust, and there have been cases where a continence adviser in an acute trust has been instructed to withdraw services from community users.

The split between providers also raises the question of who is responsible for preventive services. A Department of Health consultative report recommended that there should be a defined district budget for continence services, rather than separate budgets in different provider units, so that coordination and planning is possible for the district population as a whole (Department of Health 1991).

Respite care

The provision of respite care at the right time and in the right way can help support carers and thereby improve their quality of life, as well as prevent or delay admission to long-stay care. Health and local authorities are exhorted to provide respite care, but there are no statutory duties to do so, and there is no clear boundary between medical respite care for which health authorities are responsible, and social respite care for which local authorities are responsible. Once again this is an area which can benefit from a joint approach.

There is an example in outer London of a Night Centre which caters for people with dementia. The scheme uses transport and accommodation which are not otherwise used at night-time. The steering group includes health and social services representation, and the Centre is managed by a voluntary agency. Funding comes from joint finance and the Mental Illness Specific Grant.

Reprovision services

The challenges to collaboration of achieving reprovision of long-stay hospitals are well-documented (Knapp *et al.* 1992). Purchasers in both health and local authorities must find a way, which is acceptable to both authorities and to users, of unlocking the resources tied up in capital and medically-focused staffing, and then to transfer them to community services. In a number of areas of the country, health and local authorities have pooled their resources in a joint service for people with learning disabilities. These services are jointly planned, commissioned, resourced and monitored. Each authority contributes to the joint fund resources equivalent to what they would have otherwise been spending separately, based on previous provision and on dowry payments for people leaving long-stay hospital, and there may be substantial additions of benefit income through charges for residential care provided in independent sector hostels and group homes.

SUMMARY

While events leading from implementation of the NHS Community Care Act 1990 unfold, the structure of welfare state organizations is changing. No sooner have the health service reforms been bedded down than announcements are made to abolish Regional Health Authorities and to merge District Health Authorities and Family Health Service Authorities. And, at a time when local authorities should be giving considerable emphasis to making sure the community care changes work to the benefit of users, carers and taxpayers, the Local Government Review is throwing the plans of some county councils into turmoil and blighting others. On the provider side of the developing mixed economies of health and social care, new organizational forms and consortia are evolving to strengthen what may already be a position of considerable power and influence.

In these circumstances it would not be at all surprising if local and health authorities concentrated their attentions and energies on their own (internal) objectives, resources and expenditures. Yet, as we have argued in this chapter, the needs for, and advantages of, improved cross-agency relationships are many and various. There may be advantages in, for example, joint commissioning or joint provision, though *compatible* commissioning and provision would be a considerable step forward in many areas of the country. A small improvement would be clarity about, and dissemination of, aims and intentions, in relation to assessment and eligibility criteria, purchasing priorities, market management, quality assurance and outcome criteria.

Community care is as important to the health service as it is to local government, though it is rarely interwoven into main-stream agendas. The challenge for health service and local authority managers is to move beyond the short-term distractions of their respective health and social care implementation agendas to plan the medium- and long-term development of community care.

FURTHER READING

♦ Journals: Up-to-date material can be found in *Health Service Journal* and in *Journal of Social Policy*.

♦ Audit Commission (1986), *Making a Reality of Community Care*, HMSO, London.

♦ Knapp, M.R.J., Cambridge, P., Thomason, C., Beecham, J., Allen, C. and Darton, R. (1992), *Care in the Community: Challenge and Demonstration*, Ashgate, Aldershot.

♦ Wistow, G., Knapp, M.R.J., Hardy, B. and Allen, C. (1994), *Social Care in a Mixed Economy*, Open University Press, Buckingham.

REFERENCES

Audit Commission (1986), *Making a Reality of Community Care*. London: HMSO.

Bulmer, M. (1987), *The Social Basis of Community Care*. London: Allen & Unwin.

Challis, D., Chessum, R., Chesterman, J. *et al.* (1988), Community care for the frail elderly: an urban experiment, *British Journal of Social Work*, 18(Suppl): 13–42.

Challis, D., Chessum, R., Chesterman, J. *et al.* (1990), The Gateshead Community Care Scheme: Case Management in Social and Health Care. Canterbury: PSSRU, University of Kent.

Challis, D. and Davies, B. (1986), *Case Management in Community Care*. Aldershot: Gower.

Cmnd 849 (1989), *Caring for People*. London: HMSO.

Cmnd 6233 (1975), *Better Services for the Mentally Ill*. London: HMSO.

Davies, B. and Challis, D. (1986), *Matching Resources to Needs in Community Care*. Aldershot, Gower.

Department of Health (1991), *Agenda for Action on Continence Services*. London: HMSO.

Department of Health (1992), *Health and Personal Social Services Statistics for England*, London, HMSO.

Ernst and Whinney (1986), *Survey of Private and Voluntary Residential and Nursing Homes*. Report to the Department of Health and Social Security, London.

Farmer, R., Rolde, J. and Sachs, B. (1991), *Dimensions of Mental Handicap*, London: Charing Cross and Westminster Medical School.

Freedman, R. and Moran, A. (1984), Wanderers in a promised land: the chronically mentally ill and deinstitutionalisation, *Medical Care*, 22(Suppl):12.

Goodwin, S. (1989, Community care for the mentally ill in England and Wales: myths, assumptions and reality, *Journal of Social Policy*, 18(1):27–52.

Griffiths, R. (1988), *Community Care: Agenda for Action*. London: HMSO.

Hansard (1993), *Written Answers Col. 334*, 18 February, London: HMSO.

Harrison, L. and Means, R. (1990), *Housing: The Essential Element in Community Care*. Oxford: Anchor Housing Trust.

Henwood, M., Jowell, T. and Wistow, G. (1991), *All Things Come to Those who Wait?: Causes and Consequences of the Community Care Delays*, Briefing Paper 12. London: King's Fund Institute.

Henwood, M. and Wistow, G. (1993), The buck stops here, *Health Service Journal*, 21 October.

House of Commons Health Committee (1991), *Public Expenditure on Health and Personal Social Services*, 1, Session 1990–91, HC614-1. London: HMSO.

House of Commons Social Services Committee (1985), *Community Care*, 2, Session 1984–85, HC13. London: HMSO.

Kavanagh, S., Knapp, M.R.J., Beecham, J. and Opit, L. (1993a), The costs of schizophrenia care in England: preliminary estimates. Report to the Department of Health, Discussion Paper 920, Personal Social Services Research Unit, University of Kent at Canterbury.

Kavanagh, S., Schneider, J., Knapp, M.R.J., Beecham, J. and Netten, A. (1993b), Elderly people with cognitive impairment: costing possible changes in the balance of care, *Health and Social Care in the Community*, 1(2):69–80.

Kelly, A. (1991), The new managerialism in the social services. In: Carter P, (Ed.), *Social Work and Social Welfare Yearbook*, Vol. 3. Harlow: Longman.

Knapp, M.R.J. (1994), Community mental health services: towards an understanding of cost-effectiveness. In: Creed, F. and Tyrer, P. (Eds), *Evaluation of Community Psychiatric Services*. Cambridge: Cambridge University Press.

Knapp, M.R.J., Cambridge, P., Thomason, C., Beecham, J., Allen, C. and Darton, R. (1992), *Care in the Community: Challenge and Demonstration*. Aldershot: Ashgate.

Knapp, M.R.J. and Wistow, G. (1993a), *Welfare Pluralism and Community Care Development: The Role of Local Government and the Non-statutory Sectors in Social Welfare Services in England*. Paris: Organisation for Economic Cooperation and Development.

Knapp, M.R.J. and Wistow, G. (1993b), Joint commissioning for community care. In: *Implementing Community Care: A Slice Through Time*, Department of Health Social Services Inspectorate, London.

Lawson, R. (1993), *Toolkit on Community Care for Purchasers*. London: North East Thames Regional Health Authority.

Martin, J., Meltzer, H. and Elliot, D. (1988), *The Prevalence of Disability Among Adults*. London: HMSO.

Social Services Inspectorate (1987), *From Home Help to Home Care: An Analysis of Policy, Resourcing and Service Management*. London: HMSO.

Social Services Inspectorate (1993), *Raising the Standard: The Second Annual Report of the Chief Inspector, Social Services Inspectorate 1992/93*. London: HMSO.

Walker, A. (1982), *Community Care: The Family, the State and Social Policy*. Oxford, Blackwell.

Wertheimer, A. and Greig, R. (1993), *Report on Joint Commissioning for Community Care. Manchester: National Development Team*.

Wistow, G. (1985), Community care for the mentally handicapped: disappointing progress. In: Harrison, A. and Gretton, J. (Eds), *Health Care UK 1985* London: Policy Journals.

Wistow, G. (1991), Inter-agency perspectives. In: Morgan, J. (Ed.), *Community Care Futures: The Clivenden Debate*. London: KPMG Management Consultants.

Wistow, G. (1992), Joint planning in a new policy context, *Health Services Management*, 88(1):25–28.

Wistow, G., Knapp, M.R.J., Hardy, B. and Allen, C. (1994), *Social Care in a Mixed Economy*. Buckingham: Open University Press.

Wistow, G., Leedham, I. and Hardy, B. (1993), *A Preliminary Analysis of a Sample of English Community Care Plans*. London: Department of Health.

Wistow, G. and Manning, R. (1993), *Spending in the Personal Social Services*. Leeds: Nuffield Institute for Health.

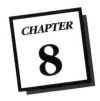

ACUTE SERVICES

Malcolm Forsythe

OBJECTIVES

- ◆ To describe the ideas and policies which have shaped the provision of acute services.

- ◆ To show how the pattern of specialist services has developed to meet epidemiological and social needs.

- ◆ To show how patterns of medical staffing and medical work have changed within the NHS.

- ◆ To examine whether the market threatens the effective provision of acute care in the NHS.

INTRODUCTION

Acute hospitals contain the most advanced, complex and expensive technologies available within health care and their management has always been the subject of debate and controversy. In themselves they represent large public capital investments and the resources they consume determine the pattern of care available to communities.

This chapter describes some of the main conceptual foundations on which the acute hospital services have developed and shows how developments in technology have changed the structure of work within them. It explains how government policies and resources have attempted to mould and develop the network of hospitals inherited from the 18th and 19th centuries which still dominate the pattern of services – as the debate over the **Tomlinson proposals** (Tomlinson *et al*. 1992) demonstrates. Changes in epidemiology and medical technology, the results of medical and health services research, and the requirements of patients, have combined to change the pattern of acute services, the nature of work in hospitals and consequently the problems faced by those who provide and manage clinical services.

THE DEVELOPMENT OF ACUTE SERVICES

Clinicians often describe the hospital system, and their own hospital in particular, as underfunded even if they are fortunate enough to be working in a newly built hospital. Even where the fabric and equipment are up to date, they are still dependent on service contracts for the necessary revenue. The **internal market** is causing important questions to be asked:

♦ How many hospitals are required?
♦ What is the optimal size of a hospital?
♦ Where should they be located?
♦ What specialties and sub-specialties should they have, and are there different types of acute hospital?

Despite attempts to clarify the role of the acute hospital the main themes can be identified in a diverse set of reports commencing soon after the First World War and demonstrating a longstanding and widespread disquiet with the role of acute services and the resources available.

The Dawson Report In 1920, the Consultative Council on Medical and Allied Services, which had been established under the Ministry of Health Act 1919, submitted an interim report on the future provision of medical and allied services. The Chairman of the Council was Lord Dawson of Penn and the report is better known today as the **Dawson Report** (Cmnd 693, 1920). The terms of reference for the report were:

> 'To consider and make recommendations as to the scheme or schemes requisite for the systematised provision of such forms of medical and allied services as should, in the opinion of the Council, be available to the inhabitants of a given area.'

The Dawson Report is still the most relevant conceptualization of the provision of health services, and is as valid today as it was in 1920, even if the labels and terms have changed somewhat. Services were divided into 'domiciliary' or 'institutional' and then into 'individual' or 'communal'.

So-called 'primary' health centres were identified as being the responsibility of general practitioners but they might also include operating, X-ray, pathological and rehabilitation facilities, and be a focal point for educational meetings. Consultants from the 'secondary' health centre, to which the primary health care is attached organizationally, but sometimes physically as well, would attend as appropriate. Preventative and curative medical services would be provided together:

> 'The Secondary health centres would receive cases referred to them by the Primary Centres either on account of difficulties of diagnosis or because in their diagnosis or treatment a highly specialised equipment was needful'.

Cases of unusual difficulty and those requiring specialized knowledge or equipment would be referred to the teaching hospitals with medical schools.

Throughout the report great emphasis is laid on:

- ♦ the interrelationship of service, teaching and research;
- ♦ a need for complete intercommunication between the different levels which would be assisted by the standardization and integration of the clinical records;
- ♦ the importance of the medical profession coming into 'organic relation with health administration'.

The report demonstrated how the latter could work by applying the principles to Gloucester and the surrounding villages. Architectural drawings of a primary health centre with inpatient and outpatient facilities were also included within the report.

Acute Services in the NHS: the 1962 plan

The Emergency Medical Service set up in the Second World War heralded the system of hospitals and health care which was to be instituted in the NHS Act in 1946. The introduction of the Region, with at least one teaching hospital within its boundaries, pointed to the development of a network of hospitals and a common planning framework.

The NHS inherited an astonishing array of hospitals, not only in terms of previous ownership but also their size, function and locality. There were a variety of specialized hospitals, particularly in relation to services for infectious diseases (including sanatoria for tuberculosis), maternity, orthopaedic, ophthalmic, ear nose and throat, psychiatry, geriatric and others.

Although there had been earlier surveys of hospitals within England and attempts to measure future needs particularly in relation to hospital beds, the first major report did not emerge until 1962 with the publication of *A Hospital Plan for England and Wales* (Cmnd 1604, 1962). The concept of the District General Hospital was introduced. It was no longer appropriate for any specialty to be providing acute care in isolation. The interdependence of one specialty on another thus became a firm feature of all future plans for acute services.

At the time of the introduction of the NHS there were thought to be, in England and Wales, 3200 hospitals with about 477 000 available beds (of which about 250 000 were acute). Just following the publication of the hospital plan there were 2234 non-psychiatric hospitals with the following size distribution:

less than 50 beds	939
50–249	989
250–499	227
500–999	75
1000+	4
Total	2234

and the bed distribution was

less than 50 beds	24 940
50–249	111 898
250–499	78 716
500–999	50 726
1000+	4 456
Total	270 736

From the above it can be seen that over 86% of hospitals contained fewer than 250 beds and that over 50% of the beds were in these hospitals. The hospital plan recommended that the district general hospitals should serve a population of between 100 and 150 thousand and that the acute aspects of all the care groups – i.e. children, adults, maternity, elderly and the mentally ill – would be treated in such hospitals which would also have a full range of outpatient, casualty and day surgical facilities. The report recommended the levels of bed provision shown in Box 8.1.

The effect of applying these norms would be that few district general hospitals would have fewer than 300 beds. The plan identified specific hospitals which would be developed by 1975. By 1966, it was necessary to produce a revised plan for a number of reasons.

Box 8.1
Recommendations for beds in the 1962 plan

◆ Acute	3.3 per 1000 population
◆ Maternity	Sufficient to fulfil the recommendations of the Committee on Maternity Services (1959) for a national average of 70% of confinements to take place in hospital, with a stay of ten days after confinement in the normal case and the provision of some seven antenatal beds per 1000 births. (This gave a national average of 0.58 beds per 1000 population in 1975, on the basis of the national projections of birth rate and population then current.)
◆ Geriatric	10 per 1000 persons aged 65 and over.
◆ Mental illness	Reducing to 1.8 per 1000 population.
◆ Mental subnormality	1.3 per 1000 population.

Firstly, and most importantly, the Minister of Health realized that beds, which determined everything else that was to be provided, were not the overriding feature of acute hospitals. Paragraph 5 stated:

'The significance of the bed as the unit for measuring the hospital provision required can be exaggerated. The quality of hospital provision can often be greatly improved and the number of inpatients treated can be increased by improving such facilities as pathology laboratories, X-ray departments, operating theatres and physiotherapy departments. Over the last ten years progress has been made in this direction, but substantial opportunities remain for improving the hospital service in this way rather than by providing additional beds. Moreover, a trend has already begun, and may be expected to grow, for those needing hospital care who would in the past have become in-patients to receive treatment as day-patients or out-patients, returning to their own homes after treatment. The domiciliary health and welfare services are increasingly able to play their part in this.'

Secondly, the report began to challenge the **normative** basis of planning on a national basis and suggested that bed needs might more appropriately be measured locally.

Finally, it was obvious that the nation did not have either the necessary construction capacity or the cash to build the district general hospitals proposed. It was also realized that improved facilities would require increased cash to run them. Although there would be fewer acute beds i.e. reduced from the existing 3.9 beds/1000 for acute in 1962 to no more than 3.0 from 1975 onwards the greater use of these beds in better designed wards would require more staff. It was forecast that £10 million a year would be required to make use of each annual investment in buildings of £73 million and that around 8000 additional staff would be taken on each year.

The relationship between the capital costs of building acute hospitals and the subsequent running costs has changed dramatically since then. Today it is estimated that a conventional hospital designed according to 'Concise' Department of Health standards would have a running cost of over £19 million from a capital investment of £61.5 million. *The fact that the annual running costs are now equivalent to one-third of the capital cost demonstrates vividly how much revenue acute hospitals consume.*

The Bonham Carter Report The 1962 hospital plan was an important part of the thinking of government and the medical profession but stood little chance of implementation as a plan of action. Indeed the 1950s had shown almost no progress in the construction of new hospitals and most doctors had to make do with the facilities that they had. It soon became clear that the 'heroic' assumptions of the hospital plan required to be revisited, and in 1966 the Central Health Services Council appointed a committee under Sir Desmond Bonham Carter 'to consider the concept of the district general hospital promulgated in 1961–62 in the light of developments since that time; and to redefine the functions which the district general hospital should perform in the health services of the future.'

The report emphasized even more the need for clinical services to be grouped together (CHSC 1969). Furthermore it was argued that no consultant should work in isolation within any acute specialty. Other factors influencing the recommendations were economies of scale, particularly in relation to the support services. It recommended an increase in the catchment population of the district general hospital to at least 200 000 and ideally 300 000 or more. This meant that the hospital could contain between 1200 and 1800 beds.

The Bonham Carter Report represented the pinnacle of the concept of a large hospital having over 1000 beds with all support services on the same site. At this time the proportion of total NHS spending devoted to hospital building had grown from less than 3% in 1951 and 4.5% in 1961 to 6.5% in 1970.

Central feature ✳

The shift towards inductive planning

The harsh economic climate in the 1970s forced everyone to rethink the basis of planning acute hospitals. The national 'deductive' or 'normative' basis of planning (i.e. number of beds, doctors, or whatever per 1000 population) was insensitive to the varying health needs in different communities. There was a distinct shift towards a bottom-up or 'inductive' approach towards identifying needs. The combination of a shortage of capital and the encouragement of local priorities in the late seventies led to some fascinating initiatives in all the care groups and encouraged greater attention being given to reduce the need for inpatient care.

Nevertheless there were still considerable geographical differences in the level of service provision for acute beds which had not been rectified by the end of the 1970s. Furthermore worldwide it had become recognized that the demand for health care was highly correlated with the level of provision. Not only were there differences in the level of provision but there were also differences to be found in hospitalization rates.

The London Health Planning Consortium was set up in 1979 to look into the hospital services within London. The profile of acute hospital services in London (LHPC 1979) not only demonstrated the effect of supply on demand but commented also on the relatively inefficient use of these beds where supply was higher. This was one of the first reports to start comparing localities using population hospitalization rates and to project future bed needs based on such rates adjusted for future population age and sex distributions and taking into account the trends in reductions in length of stay.

One of the most significant influences in the development of acute services during this period has been changes in epidemiology.

These changes are sometimes dramatic attracting widespread attention and new funding as was the case in the development of AIDS services. In other cases they begin with small changes in disease patterns and the resulting piecemeal service developments add up to significant changes in direction over a period of years. Some of these changes are examined in the next section.

EPIDEMIOLOGICAL CHANGES

The most dramatic changes have been in relation to *infectious diseases*. Sanatoria or chest hospitals for treating tuberculosis were closed down or temporarily converted for other uses. Infectious disease hospitals have been closed except for a handful of mothballed hospitals nationwide which can be opened at very short notice to deal with the very rare viral haemorrhagic diseases, such as lassa fever and Marburg disease. In December 1977, the Global Commission for the Certification of Smallpox Eradication declared the world free of smallpox and this was ratified by the World Health Assembly in May 1980.

Infectious diseases have not gone away. Indeed during the last two decades there have been a number of new infectious diseases (e.g. HIV/AIDS, listeriosis, legionnaires disease) which have created a need for inpatient care. The difference is that isolation is far less important than being properly treated in an acute hospital where all the appropriate diagnostic and therapeutic services are available. In addition, there are now many more patients who are at great risk of infection as a result of being treated by particular immunosuppressive drugs or radiotherapy treatment. These patients may require the most stringent precautions being taken to prevent being harmed by organisms which are otherwise of little harm to a person whose immune system is functioning properly.

One could not leave the subject of infectious diseases without reflecting on the problems which may beset any community which has achieved herd immunity for normal children's infectious diseases but where the immunization programme collapses. Diseases such as whooping cough, polio, diphtheria and measles, which have not been abolished, can cause even more severe morbidity in adults who become infected. Recent events in Russia have provided a vivid demonstration of this in relation to diphtheria. There could be a massive requirement for acute inpatient facilities which might be difficult to meet.

Many *chronic physical diseases* have also changed in relation to their incidence and prevalence. Morris (1979) describes how in Victorian England, peptic ulcer commonly took the form of acute gastric ulcer in young women, a condition rarely seen nowadays. He goes on to describe the way in which duodenal ulcers reached epidemic proportions in the 1930s and 1940s but have been receding since the 1950s. Perforation of the gut wall or severe bleeding were all very serious conditions requiring emergency admission into hospital. For those for whom medical treatment was incapable of providing relief, some form of surgery was the only alternative. Morris estimated that between 1953 and 1959 about 20 000 elective operations for ulcer were done annually on men of which two-thirds were for duodenal ulcer. Today there is an effective medical therapy, particularly for those patients with a peptic ulcer in whom *Helicobacter pylorii* is cultured, for whom a complete cure can be expected from drug treatment alone.

The treatment of *mental health* has also changed dramatically the need for hospital beds. Apart from acute facilities in the general hospital, it is now common to find most other services provided in the community. Patients suffering from substance abuse may only need to be detoxified in the hospital.

SPECIALIST SERVICES

The relationship between volume and quality

When the Health Sub-Committee of the US Senate visited the United Kingdom in 1971, it was particularly complimentary about the family practitioner services – not just for what they provided but also for how they helped to avoid encumbering the hospital services with minor complaints more appropriately dealt with by the primary care team (US Senate 1971). The other major achievement identified by the visiting US team was the way in which the specialist services had become more rationally and equitably provided. The combined benefit of these features was that the UK managed to provide its health services with fewer neurosurgeons than were practising in San Francisco. This observation raised the possibilities not only that there were more of those specialists than were justified on workload terms, but also that the experience gained by each was possibly insufficient to maintain a satisfactory level of clinical expertise.

The relationship between volume and outcome is extremely complex. The whole training programme in medicine is designed to emphasize the importance of apprenticeship in order to achieve sufficient practice before being allowed to work independently as a specialist. This point has been strengthened during the last 25 years by the development of continuing medical education and the need constantly to update knowledge within the relevant field.

Dramatic changes in diagnostic and therapeutic procedures during the last decade (e.g. keyhole surgery and minimally invasive procedures under radiological viewing) have highlighted the fact that it is not necessarily sufficient to be registered as a specialist and attend regular updating, but that to undertake some of these new procedures, it is necessary firstly to be taught and then to practise under supervision by an expert before returning to do this work unsupervised. This method has recently been adopted by the Royal College of Surgeons of England as a result of new evidence pointing to increased mortality and morbidity in new techniques where there had been insufficient training and experience. Deaths were

*New
technologies
Medical
Audit

↑ Death
Rates*

being reported in patients who would not have been expected to die with conventional surgery. This has been identified as a result of increased surveillance and clinical audit.

Luft *et al*. (1990) have looked carefully at the literature on the relationship between volume and quality. They have described another possible relationship – namely that if someone is regarded as an expert with good results, then more cases will be referred. This is usually referred to as '**selective referral**'.

Comparisons of hospital results may mask variable performance of specialists. Box 8.2 shows standardized hospital death rates for elective (planned) and emergency patients operated on for aortic aneurysms. Although there were differences between Kent hospi-

Box 8.2
Example of how
surgeon performance
variations are masked

Standardized hospital death ratios (SETRHA standard = 100) for operated aneurysms in Kent hospitals, 1988–1993

	Emergencies	Electives
Kent	96 (82–111)	110 (80–148)
Hospital		
William Harvey	100	60
Buckland	107	150
Thanet	108	114
Kent and Canterbury	91	112
Joyce Green	96	83
Maidstone	100	50
Medway	136	86
Kent and Sussex	100	400

All surgeons who did <20 operations against all those who did 20 or more operations

	Total number of operations	Deaths	Survivors
Surgeons (*N* = 19) who did <20 elective and emergency selected operations	127	61 (**48%**)	66 (**52%**)
Surgeons (*N* = 19) who did 20 or more elective and emergency selected operations	760	166 (**22%**)	594 (**78%**)

tals and Kent as a whole compared with the rest of the South East Thames Regional Health Authority, none of these were significant. On the other hand, when the *surgeons* were divided up into those who did less than 20 operations within six years and those who did more, then the differences in the mortality rate of those operated on *were* significantly different (chi-squared significance at 1% level).

There may also be questions to be answered about the effect on quality in relation to experience over time or scale of numbers at any time. A hospital which has treated many cases over many years can be expected to have the best possible results. However, the number of cases necessary either over time or within a year will vary according to the condition or treatment, and some new risks may occur when a unit becomes too large (e.g. possible increase in cross-infections or the staff may become frustrated as a result of the monotony of doing the same work repeatedly). This is why most surgeons like to have a variety of cases on operation lists and why very few hospitals are keen to repeat weeks dedicated to only one operation (e.g. hernias or cataracts) in order to relieve waiting lists.

There are hospitals which specialize in undertaking specific procedures only (e.g. terminations or joint replacements) but on the whole they are exceptional. Much greater importance is now given to creating centres for treating sufficient workload to enable a team of four or more specialists to undertake the full range of duties within a specialty and provide a continuous service all year round. This has been a marked feature of designated supra-regional and regional services in the past; although even more progress might have been made if adequate documentation on the relationship between volume and outcome had been available to convince the public and politicians alike within a community that rationalization was in their interests even if it was at the expense of increased travelling.

The interdependence of specialists has been increasing steadily over time. This has to some extent been exacerbated by the huge increase in specialties. The list below shows the number of new specialties recognized within general medicine since 1979. There are now 55 specialties listed in the Department of Health breakdown of hospital specialties (DoH 1993a).

Old-age psychiatry	1979
Clinical genetics	1979
Paediatric neurology	1980
Rheumatology	1982
Occupational health	1983
Thoracic medicine	1984
Palliative medicine	1989
Clinical cytogenetics	1989
Virology	1989
Rehabilitation	1990
Clinical immunology and allergy	1990

It is not untypical to see patterns of care develop which automatically pass the management of patients from one consultant to another. The most common example is perhaps joint replacement in the elderly, particularly following fracture of the neck of the femur. Recently an expert advisory group on *cancer* to the Chief Medical Officers of England (DoH 1994) proposed three levels of care:

- There would be the main focus of care.
- There would be designated cancer units of a size to support clinical teams with sufficient expertise and facilities to manage the commoner cancers (e.g. breast, lung and gastrointestinal), with multidisciplinary consultation and management.
- There would be the cancer centre which would treat 'the less common and rare cancers and those treatment regimes which are too specialized, technically demanding or capital intensive to be provided in the secondary centre.'

While it cannot be said that the development of the specialist services has been built upon these findings, there is evidence of development and adjustment to meet many of the fundamental assumptions outlined above.

Regional specialties The creation of the regional hospital structure in 1948 was particularly valuable for the development and control of those services which demanded particular skills in diagnosis and/or treatment or which were too uneconomic to provide in every district general hospital.

During the 1970s, the concept of the regional provision of services became prevalent worldwide and the source of considerable envy in those countries which were unable to organize them in this way. Kerr-White argued (in Saward 1975) that the principal reason for regionalization was related to patient problems and was epidemiological in nature. He described three types of epidemiological problem. The first relates to common ailments which are appropriate at the primary care level. Then there are those which are appropriate at the secondary care level, and finally those requiring populations of

'a half million to a million or so to generate sufficient numbers to really occupy and maintain the skills of the tertiary care levels, the supporting staff and the necessary technological facilities and equipment'.

In 1976, the government consulted on priorities for health and personal social services (DHSS 1976). On general and acute hospital services, mention is made of the trend towards greater and greater interdependence of the various branches of medicine and the growing need to bring together a wide range of facilities for diagnosis and treatment. There was still the problem of services for conditions which were so rare as to require consideration at a national level.

Supra-regional services In 1983, a Supra-Regional Services Advisory Group was set up to advise the Secretary of State through the chairmen of regional health authorities on the identification of services to be funded supra-regionally and on the appropriate level of provision (DoH 1992/93). The group established the criteria shown in Box 8.3 for selecting services.

Box 8.3
Criteria for services to be funded supra-regionally

♦ The service should be an established clinical service, not a research or development activity (for which alternative sources of funding exist).

♦ There should be a clearly defined group of patients having a clinical need for the service.

♦ The benefits of the service should be sufficient to justify its costs when set against alternative uses of NHS funds.

♦ The cost should be high enough to make the service a significant burden for the providing regions.

♦ Supra-regional funding, as opposed to regional or sub-regional development, should be clearly justified either
(a) by the small number of potential patients in relation to the minimal viable workload for a centre, or
(b) by the economic and service benefits of concentrating the service in fewer and larger units shared between regions (this does not include services organized mainly at regional level in which two regions agree on joint provision as a matter of mutual convenience), or
(c) as an interim measure, by the scarcity of the relevant expertise and/or facilities.

♦ The units to be designated should be capable of meeting the total national caseload for England and Wales.

In the first year about ten services were recognized, and each year a review was to be made of new proposals submitted and the question of retaining existing services. In 1992/93 contracts totalling over £89 million were agreed by the Department of Health with the designated units for the 13 services shown in Box 8.4. However, the government has now decided to devolve this service since it conflicts with the internal market.

Box 8.4
Supra-regional services
funded in 1992/93

Designated service	Contract value (£millions)	Percentage share
Choriocarcinoma	1.4	1.5
Craniofacial service	2.3	2.6
Fulminant hepatic failure	2.1	2.4
Heart transplantation	23.8	26.7
Liver transplantation	18.0	20.2
Neonatal and infant cardiac surgery	25.2	28.2
Paediatric liver disease	5.6	6.2
Primary bone tumour	6.0	6.7
Psychiatric services for the deaf	3.0	3.3
Retinoblastoma	0.9	1.0
Stereotactic radiosurgery	0.5	0.5
Proton treatment of uveal melanomas	0.5	0.5
Total	89.1	100.0

CHANGING PATTERNS OF CARE WITHIN HOSPITALS

In the past, patients admitted to open Nightingale-type wards would usually stay there until discharge. Seriously ill patients were located close to the nurses' station, and the day room was furthest away together with the fittest patients. For some conditions, patients may have been transferred to a preconvalescent ward and/or convalescent unit before returning to their normal place of residence.

The creation of more privacy by providing 4- and 6-bed bays and more single and double rooms, together with more stringent fire regulations, created major problems for patient observation and care. This created the need for patients to be classified as high, medium or low dependency, often with the aid of a computerized nurse dependency system. The 1960s and 1970s saw the introduction of Intensive Care Units, first of all dealing with all types of acutely ill patients but increasingly moving towards specialized units (e.g. coronary care). Patients recovering from surgery would remain close to the theatre in a recovery area and would not be returned to the ward until conscious. Many accident patients requiring observation would be accommodated in an accident ward overnight and then either admitted to a proper ward the next day or discharged. Patients recovering from a stroke would be transferred after early treatment to a stroke rehabilitation unit. Those admitted with a fractured neck of femur would be transferred postoperatively into an ortho-geriatric rehabilitation unit.

The last two decades, therefore, have seen patient transfers within hospitals increasing rapidly. Preconvalescent wards and convalescent hospitals have virtually disappeared, but there has

[handwritten margin note: Possible Return of Local Hosp following surgery]

been a great deal of interest lately in the concept of a local hospital to treat patients still requiring nursing and rehabilitation once they no longer need to be in the acute hospital.

It is hardly surprising that some efforts have been made recently to stop moving patients around the hospital – whether to other wards or to departments for investigation and/or treatment – and develop forms of patient-based care when everything possible is done to bring services to the patient. Clearly there are some services that can be provided at the bedside and it is possible to extend the skills of care staff treating patients to reduce multiple handling. The benefits to the patients and the effects on staff and on the costs of these schemes (e.g. patient focused or centred care) have not yet been identified.

Another development which has had significant effect on acute hospitals and the work they do relates to *terminal care*. Box 8.5 shows the place of death of people since 1974.

Box 8.5
Where people died within England and Wales (percentages)

Year	Home	Hospital and other establishments for the care of the sick		Other
		NHS	*Non-NHS*	
1974	37 (31 own home)	56	3	4
1983	33	58	4	5
1990	28	55	10	7
1991	27 (23 own home)	54	11	8

In 1991, there were 570 044 deaths

The deceased's home or a relative's home is continuing to diminish in importance as the place of death. Indeed over 70% of deaths were at home at the beginning of the century; in 1991 this had decreased to 27% with 23% being in the deceased's own home. There has been a trebling in the percentage of deaths in non-NHS hospitals and communal establishments for the care of the sick. A considerable portion of this is due to the rapid expansion of the hospices (most of which are outside the NHS). The number of hospice beds has increased from 1000 in 1972 to over 3000 in 1992. In addition to the expansion of hospices, there has also been a huge increase in non-NHS nursing home provision, which care for many patients who would previously have been in long-stay NHS beds for the elderly, the mentally ill and those with learning disabilities. Community care has also encouraged the development of sheltered housing which helps to account for the increase in deaths in the 'other' category.

Hospices traditionally care for patients with cancers and other conditions requiring skills in symptom and pain control. Such patients previously died either at home or in hospital. The reduction in such deaths in hospitals has been offset by deaths for other conditions which previously might not have been treated in hospital.

There are some emergency conditions for which it is important to seek admission to hospital as soon as possible. The most important of these numerically is acute myocardial infarction, where 30% of deaths occur instantly and around 45% within two hours. Efforts are being made to reduce the 'pain (or the attack) to treatment time' by developing ways to fast track admission to the coronary care unit or to deliver specialized medical treatment to the patient at home as quickly as possible. Ambulances will soon all have trained paramedics on board able to undertake cardiopulmonary resuscitation and other critical treatment. Developments with telemetry are also enabling expert opinions to be provided over long distances. This brings us to a consideration of one of the key distinguishing features of acute hospitals through which many of the patient and support services are driven.

Accident and emergency departments

An interesting feature of the NHS has been the steady increase in emergency admissions. Allegations have been made that this is as a result of the introduction of contracting. Thus hospitals on a cost-volume contract may be unable to receive any more non-emergencies within the financial year as the contract has been fulfilled. Other explanations have suggested abuse by general practitioner fundholders who do not have to reimburse the hospital service for emergency treatment. Additionally, non-GP fundholders might be able to secure an admission to a particular hospital for which the health authority does not have a contract.

A great deal of attention is being given in many countries to the improvement of Accident and Emergency (A and E) departments, particularly in relation to quality standards. Whilst an acute hospital can exist without an accident and emergency department, the latter cannot exist without being located in a hospital which has certain core specialties available on site. These are identified in Box 8.6.

Around 20% of patients attending an accident and emergency department are admitted. Many are kept for observation only and so it is quite common for there to be an observation ward and in some hospitals an admission ward. Patients then may be discharged the next morning or admitted into a specialist ward.

Such a critical mass of staff and facilities cannot be justified unless there is sufficient workload. There is general support that a unit should have at least 25 000 new cases a year, and ideally 35 000 and not more than 90–100 thousand at the maximum. In urban areas the minimum size might appropriately be raised to 50 000 new cases.

Box 8.6
Access to specialties
from A & E

It is standard now to expect inpatient facilities in the following specialties in any 24-hour department (Department of Health 1993b, SE Thames RHA 1994):

General medicine
General surgery
Paediatrics
Trauma and orthopaedics
Obstetrics and gynaecology
Anaesthetics

In addition there must be adequate provision of intensive care and coronary care beds. There must be access within half an hour to a range of other specialties including:

ENT
Ophthalmology
Psychiatry
Geriatrics
Neurosurgery and neurology
Maxillo-facial
Plastic surgery and burns
Paediatric
Cardiothoracic

Certain support departments are critical, including a fully staffed operating theatre available 24 hours a day for emergencies, on-site X-ray including computerized tomography, and pathology including a mortuary.

Many patients attending an A & E department will require minimal treatment and will return home. Many experiments have been devised to see how primary care type cases can be best dealt with – including locating casualty facilities within a health centre, a local community hospital, or even providing a primary care unit within an A & E department. Ideally there should be some functional integration between all units providing emergency services and this can be strengthened by having protocols agreed by all concerned. Peripheral minor injury or casualty units should not receive any ambulance cases. They may be staffed by doctors and nurses or just nurse practitioners.

The ambulance service, which brings non-ambulant emergencies to hospital, is becoming increasingly sophisticated. By the end of 1995, all front-line vehicles will have a paramedic on board trained in skills such as airway management, the insertion of a cannula into a vein, cardiac resuscitation and monitoring, and administration of certain drugs. Monitoring is becoming increasingly sophisticated as a result of telemetry. A consequence of these increased skills is that more patients may be diagnosed before reaching hospital, thus enabling direct admission to units such as coronary care where the earliest possible treatment may be critical to their short- and long-term benefit.

Acute hospitals without an accident and emergency department can still receive emergency admissions when the patients have been referred by a general practitioner and accepted in advance by the hospital. Such patients would be seen in an independent admissions unit.

Experiments are being undertaken to measure the effectiveness of regional trauma units serving at least a million population. Benefits of such units have been described in other countries. Such units would be expected to have on site those specialties listed in Box 8.6 as being only within close access of an A & E department.

Many conurbations have too many A & E departments, and because it is regarded as a critical facility to enhance and maintain the hospital's future for care, teaching and research, there is often great reluctance to reduce them. Some hospitals have negotiated rosters for being on call on different days, nights or weekends, but this is regarded as a very unsatisfactory compromise which is wasteful in resources and potentially dangerous for patients.

To Many A+E Depts

CHANGING PATTERNS OF WORK WITHIN HOSPITALS

The dramatic improvements in diagnostic and therapeutic techniques, coupled with a consistent drive to improve efficiency and provide care in the most appropriate way, have all affected the need for hospital beds. Hospitals have closed involving all specialties.

Figure 8.1 shows the changes in hospitals and beds between 1959 and 1991. Initially most of the closures related to single specialty hospitals – maternity, infectious disease, ENT etc. Then during the 1980s there began the closures of hospitals for those with learning difficulties (previously 'mentally handicapped'), mentally ill and the elderly. These all reflected a shift from hospital to community care for these services. It was originally intended that the acute aspects of caring for the elderly, elderly mentally ill and the mentally ill would be accommodated on the acute hospital site, but while this still pertains for the elderly, alternative models are promoted for the other two services.

The Audit Commission (1990) highlighted the waste of NHS resources as a result of patients being treated as inpatients for conditions which could be undertaken as day cases. The government now publishes data on the degree to which hospitals undertake day surgery as a proportion of the total surgical workload. Already there are hospitals achieving over 60% day-case work

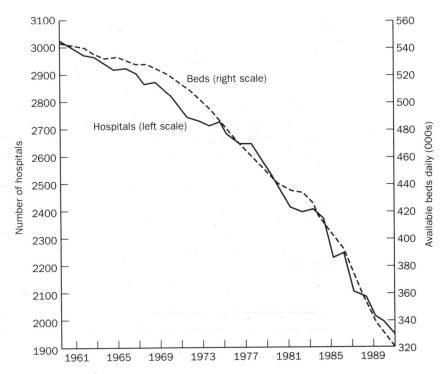

Figure 8.1
Number of NHS hospitals and daily average available beds in the UK
(Source: *Office of Health Economics Compendium of Health Statistics*, 7th edn 1992)

and it may not be ridiculous to contemplate the figure reaching 80%.

Box 8.7 shows the ten most common conditions for admission into acute hospitals in 1980 and 1991. The sudden appearance of asthma in 1991 as the second most common condition reflects a real increase. Although the death rate for myocardial infarction is falling, the discharges and deaths from hospital have risen reflecting the policy of admitting all cases as quickly as possible. Cerebrovascular diseases reflect the changing age structure of the population.

Another way of looking at the use of beds is in relation to the number used daily by those leading causes, as shown in Box 8.8. Thus cerebrovascular disease is the most significant condition, using two and a half times the number of beds of the next commonest, pneumonia. Although there was a 30% increase in discharge for strokes between 1980 and 1991, there was a drop in the number of beds used in the time period. It is interesting to see how the five most common causes for bed use in 1980 remain the five commonest causes in 1991, still covering over 20% of all the beds used.

Box 8.7
Number of NHS
hospital discharges
and deaths by leading
causes (England)

(Thousands)	1980		1991
All causes	4468		5883
Abortion	109	Abdominal pain (ill-	
Cerebrovascular disease	107	defined condition)	167
Abdominal pain (ill-		Asthma	149
defined condition)	103	Cerebrovascular disease	134
Hernia of abdominal		Acute myocardial	
cavity	99	infarction	132
Acute myocardial		Abortion	123
infarction	90	Hernia of abdominal	
Chronic disease of tonsils		cavity	99
and adenoids	76	Cataract	79
Teeth and supporting		Teeth and supporting	
structures	63	structures	77
Appendicitis	59	Rheumatism, excluding	
Menstrual disorders	54	the back	66
Pneumonia	52	Pneumonia	60
Malignant neoplasm of			
trachea, bronchus and			
lung	52		

Source: *Hospital In-Patient Enquiry, Office of Health Economics Compendium of Health Statistics*, 1992

Box 8.8
Distribution of NHS
hospital beds used
daily by leading causes
(England)

(Percentage)	1980		1991
Cerebrovascular		Cerebrovascular	
disease	11.1	disease	10.3
Pneumonia	3.9	Pneumonia	4.0
Fracture of neck of		Osteoarthrosis and allied	
femur	2.6	disorders	2.4
Osteoarthrosis and allied		Fracture of neck of	
disorders	2.1	femur	2.2
Acute myocardial		Acute myocardial	
infarction	2.1	infarction	2.1

Source: *Hospital In-Patient Enquiry, Office of Health Economics Compendium of Health Statistics*, 1992

Box 8.9
Average length of stay
in NHS hospitals by
leading causes
(England)

(Days)	1980		1991
All causes	12.4		8.62
Cerebrovascular disease	57.5	Cerebrovascular disease	39.7
Pneumonia	40.9	Pneumonia	35.7
Fracture of neck of femur	37.5	Fracture of neck of femur	23.8
Rheumatoid arthritis except spine	36.4	Osteoarthrosis and allied disorders	21.8
Osteoarthrosis and allied disorders	31.8	Diabetes mellitus	17.2

Source: as Box 8.7

Box 8.10
Number of surgical
operations in NHS
hospitals (England)

(Thousands)	1980		1991
All operations	2206		2574
D&C/biopsy	127	Treatment of fracture by operations	124
Tonsils and adenoids	94	D&C/biopsy	120
Treatment of fracture by operations	87	Cystoscopy (with destruction of lesion)	90
Cystoscopy (with destruction of lesion)	83	Other teeth, gums and jaws	89
Inguinal hernia	71	Other operations on stomach	88

Source: as Box 8.7

Box 8.9 shows the five main conditions with the longest length of stay. For all causes during the interval, the average length of stay has dropped over 30%. The appearance of diabetes is a reflection of the length of stay for other conditions dropping more, as in 1980 the average length of stay for this condition was 18.2 days.

An analysis of surgical operations in the same period (Box 8.10) shows an increase of over 16%. The inclusion of 'other operations on the stomach' reflects the major increase in endoscopy work.

Information sources

In the 1960s the most that would be found in relation to computerization would have embraced payroll, basic accounting and some analytical processing work within laboratories, X-ray and radiotherapy departments. Data on the patients treated would usually be transferred from a coding sheet to a computer bureau. Now within many hospitals, there are integrated computer systems connecting the main patient administrative system with other application areas, embracing clinical service departments (e.g. theatres, X-ray, pathology) and other support services (e.g. pharmacy, personnel, finance). Hospitals are increasingly connected directly with purchasing authorities and general practices.

+'s with intro of I.T.

The quality of clinical information has improved dramatically since the NHS reforms of 1991. Hospitals which wished to become self-governing trusts had to demonstrate that they had developed resource management systems which included case-mix data, thus enabling clinical budgeting to be developed. Experience has shown that general practitioner fundholders and purchasing authorities are not prepared to accept incomplete information, particularly for extracontractual referrals. However, there is still no integrated personal health record nationwide and a great deal of work remains to be done to produce a clinical information system which can separate out the complexity and severity of one case from another. The **Read Codes** will be introduced shortly in the NHS and, if implementation is successful, it could be a very important step forward.

The developments discussed above have only been possible because of very significant changes in the types of staff available within and employed by the NHS.

CLINICAL MANPOWER IN THE NHS

There have been some astonishing changes to the number and distribution of people working within the NHS, the majority of whom work within the hospital service. Figure 8.2 shows, for all NHS staff, the changes to the various categories relative to a baseline figure in 1980. All categories have increased – nurses and midwives by less than 10%, compared with the professional staff group which includes professions allied to medicine, professional and scientific, and professional and technical staff with their near 40% increase.

The actual number of people employed by the hospitals fell during the 1980s by 1% (see Box 8.11), but the fall was mainly in works and ancillary staff and arose as a result of the competitive tendering development, which resulted in many hospitals contracting out for these services. This may change with an increase in success of inhouse tenders and the protected terms and conditions of service affecting staff transferred to non-NHS organizations.

In order to help reduce the burden on junior doctors, and the government's intentions to develop a consultant-based rather than consultant-led service, the policy in the decade from 1980 to 1990 was to increase the number of consultants by 2.5% a year. This has by and large been achieved as can be seen from Box 8.12. There have, however, been considerable variations between

Figure 8.2
Staff employed directly
by the NHS in the UK

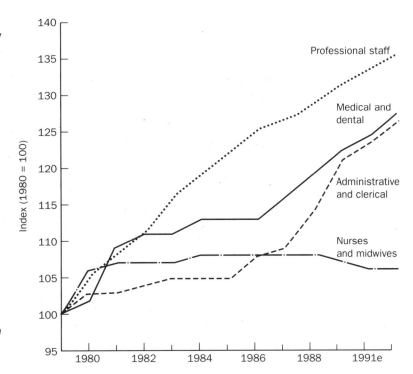

(Source: *Office of Health
Economics Compendium
of Health Statistics*, 7th
edn 1992)

	1980	% total	1990	% total	1980–1990 % change
Hospital medical & dental	35 850	5	42 870	6	+20
Hospital nursing staff	308 815	43	328 056	46	+6
Hospital midwifery	17 163	2	19 689	3	+15
Professional & technical	61 893	8	83 987	12	+36
Works	5 931	1	3 902	1	−34
Maintenance	20 572	3	16 019	2	−22
Administrative & clerical	101 786	14	125 714	17	+24
Ancillary	171 893	24	95 251	13	−46
Total	723 903	100	715 488	100	−1

Box 8.11
Balance of hospital staff numbers (whole-time equivalents) in 1980 and 1990 (England)

	1981	% total	1991	% total	1980–1990 % change
Consultants/specialists					
Anaesthetics	1529	14	2072	14	+35
Mental illness	963	8	1106	8	+13
General medicine	886	8	1138	8	+28
General surgery	836	7	911	6	+9
Radiology	774	7	1120	8	+45
Obstetrics/gynaecology	627	6	745	5	+19
Trauma/orthopaedics	598	5	733	5	+23
Histopathology	464	4	548	4	+18
Paediatrics	448	4	723	5	+61
Geriatrics	391	3	512	3	+31
Others	3832	34	4894	34	+28
Totals	11348	100	14502	100	+28
General medical practitioners					
Principals all	22518		25824		+15

Box 8.12
Analysis of hospital medical staff by specialty (England) (DoH 1993a)

the specialties. Anaesthetics remains the largest specialty – which has been brought on not just by the increase in surgical specialties requiring anaesthetic assistance, but also because of their active interest in intensive care and the development of pain control services particularly for the terminally ill.

Radiology continues its huge expansion, particularly as a result of its involvement in non-invasive interventional work, and new imaging techniques.

Perhaps one of the most radical changes which has taken place within the hospital service relates to the creation of the healthcare assistant grade, which is paid on the Administrative and Clerical Pay Scales. Essentially the post can be deployed where a task needs performing for which staff can be trained but do not necessarily need to be qualified. It has always been a matter of concern within the NHS that even for the most trivial tasks it was necessary to employ professional staff. Within every professional activity there are many tasks for which one does not really require the full qualification. During the last 25 years a lot of progress has been made to extend the role of some professional staff, particularly nursing, but there had been no sweeping proposal which could be applied to any current professional tasks which might be performed, after training, by an unqualified person. This development was introduced by the NHSME (now NHSE) at a time when there were a number of departments of acute hospitals which were notoriously difficult to staff and yet which were critical to functioning (e.g. operating theatres, A & E, X-ray and pathology departments). Since this grade has been introduced, there have been some very innovative schemes developed.

The creation of self-governing hospital and community trusts has also opened up new opportunities for employing staff in different ways. The concept of contracts with tenure until retirement is likely to change, although it is far from clear what the ideal contract would be. Pay and other terms and conditions of service can all be determined locally by trusts when taking on new staff.

The combined effect of the creation of an unqualified grade to undertake tasks previously performed by professional staff and the ability of hospital trusts to employ staff on their own terms creates the situation whereby the government can abandon the amazingly complex **Whitley Council** machinery and the review bodies set up to recommend to governments the pay of most professional NHS staff.

PRIVATE PROVISION

At the end of 1991, it was estimated that about 6.5 million people were insured for private hospital care. This represents about 11.0% of the population. The income raised from premiums amounted to some £1.4 billion in 1991, which is equivalent to about 3.5% of total health care expenditure.

The geographical distribution of privately insured people is not known but the location of private hospitals treating acute cases clearly reflects the demand for such services. There is a distinct gradient from north to south, with the South East of England having the largest provision.

Most work undertaken in these hospitals is elective surgery and estimates have been made that around 30% of elective surgery in the South East is undertaken privately. Clearly this represents a huge bonus or subsidy to the NHS purchasers within the high-uptake area. Williams and Nichol (1994) have demonstrated that in 1992/3, private hospitals admitted 429 172 inpatients and 249 531 day cases which represented respectively 7% and 154% more than in 1986. Some 5% of cases were under NHS contracts.

Despite the increased provision and use of private hospitals, they have massive spare capacity through having only 48% bed occupancy.

SUMMARY

Despite changing disease incidence and prevalence, many innovative diagnostic services and treatments, and the massive reduction in inpatient provision, the principles outlined in 1920 remain fundamentally the same. To ensure the best quality of care, there must be some hierarchical arrangement which ensures patients are treated at the appropriate level. An improvement in health services can only be achieved by a careful balancing of service provision, education and training, and research.

If the market damages this intricate system of interrelationships then it is likely that inefficiencies will enter the national health care system so that the quality of services and outcomes will be adversely affected. At the centre of the dilemma are those clinicians increasingly called upon to take up demanding roles, such as medical and clinical directors. The management of such an important system also falls increasingly heavily on the individual clinician, who will increasingly have not only to master a rapidly developing specialism but also to be adept at operating in a complex managerial environment.

FURTHER READING

♦ Journals: Up-to-date research on the management of acute health services is reported in the *British Medical Journal*.

♦ Audit Commission (1990), *A Short Cut to Better Services: Day Surgery in England and Wales*, HMSO, London.

♦ Chief Medical Officers (1994), *Policy Framework for Commissioning Cancer Services*, Department of Health, London.

♦ Ministry of Health (1990), *Interim Report on the Future Provision of Medical and Allied Services* (Chairman: Lord Dawson of Penn), Cmnd 1604, HMSO, London.

REFERENCES

Audit Commission (1990), *A Short Cut to Better Services: Day Surgery in England and Wales*. London: HMSO.

Central Health Services Council (1969), *The Functions of the District General Hospital* (the Bonham Carter Report). London: HMSO.

Cmnd 693 (1920), *Interim Report on the Future Provision of Medical and Allied Services: Consultative Council on Medical and Allied Services* (Chairman Lord Dawson of Penn). London: HMSO.

Cmnd 1604 (1962), *A Hospital Plan for England and Wales*. London: HMSO.

Department of Health and Social Security (1976), *Priorities for Health and Personal Social Services in England: A Consultative Document*. London: HMSO.

Department of Health (1992/93), *Supra Regional Services Advisory Group Annual Report*. London: HMSO.

Department of Health (1993a), *Health and Personal Social Services Statistics for England*. London: HMSO.

Department of Health (1993b), *A & E Services in London: An Initial Review of Services for the Inner London Purchasing Authorities*. Department of Health circular.

Department of Health (1994), *Policy Framework for Commissioning Cancer Services* – consultative document prepared by an expert advisory group on cancer to the Chief Medical Officers of England & Wales, May 1994 (circular).

London Health Planning Consortium (1979), *Acute Hospital Services in London - A Profile*. London: HMSO.

Luft, H.S., Garnick, D.W., Mark, D.H. and McPhee, S.J. (1990), *Hospital Volume, Physician Volume, and Patient Outcomes: Assessing the Evidence*. Ann Arbor: Health Administration Press Perspectives.

Morris, J.N. (1979), *Uses of Epidemiology*. Edinburgh: Churchill Livingstone.

Saward, E.W. (Ed.) (1975), *The Regionalization of Personal Health Services*. London: Millbank Memorial Fund, Prodist.

South East Thames Regional Health Authority (1994), *Standards for Accident and Emergency Services - Revised Edition*. London: SETRHA.

Tomlinson, B. *et al.* (1992), *Report of the Enquiry into London's Health Service*, Medical Education and Research. London: HMSO.

US Senate (1971), *Report of Visit to the United Kingdom of the US Senate Health Sub Committee*.

Williams, B.T. and Nicholl, J.P. (1994), Patient characteristics and clinical caseload of short stay independent hospitals in England and Wales, 1992-3, *BMJ*, 308: 1699-701.

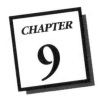

PATIENTS AS CONSUMERS

CHAPTER 9

Michael Calnan

OBJECTIVES

> ◆ To show how attention to consumer interests has become an important issue for providers of health care.
>
> ◆ To examine the impact of government policies such as charterism and complaints procedures.
>
> ◆ To examine issues of choice and quality from the consumer's perspective.

INTRODUCTION

Over the last 20 years the issue of consumerism within health care has never been far from the political agenda. However, it has been the focus of attention for a variety of reasons and it is possible to identify a range of contexts in which it has been discussed.

◆ First, increasing emphasis has been placed on the *quality* of health care and there has been a growing recognition that a comprehensive assessment of health care should take into account not only cost-effectiveness and efficiency but also include consumer opinions about health and health care. Thus, it has been argued that evaluations of health care should focus not only upon measures of clinical effectiveness and economic efficiency but also upon indicators of social acceptability to the consumers of health care.

◆ Second, with the shift from acute to chronic forms of disease in late 20th century western society, coupled with changes in the age structure of the population, issues concerning the quality of long-term medical and social care come to the fore. With chronic forms of disease and disability, sufferers and their families play a more active part in management of treatment and care.

◆ Third, consumer satisfaction may be important not only as an outcome variable in its own right but also as a mediating variable which may influence, amongst other things, treatment 'compliance' – which in turn might influence health status and medical outcomes.

◆ The fourth context relates to the realm of political beliefs. That is to say, some have argued that taking the views and opinions of consumers or citizens into account – such as through increased 'participation' in the policy-making or decision-making process – may serve as a means of democratizing health services, thus making both the medical profession and the state more accountable. Alternatively, others have emphasized a somewhat different political philosophy, concerned with issues of 'consumer sovereignty' and the need for healthcare systems to be tailored to meet the demands and choices of its customers. This tends to focus on individual demands although with the shift from 'implicit' to 'explicit' rationing, increasingly the 'public' and 'community' are being asked for their views about priorities in the provision of health care. The UK's government has encouraged commissioning health authorities to listen to 'local voices', although emphasis is placed on being responsive rather than on active community participation.

♦ The fifth context relates to the realm of professional ethics and humanitarian concerns. The emphasis here is placed upon the altruistic concern of the doctor with the patient's welfare. For example, some doctors emphasize the holistic nature of therapeutic care, which by definition requires that the concerns and interests of the patient be taken into account. Also, in the context of ethics some professionals emphasize the need to inform patients about the risks of different treatments or medical interventions and leave the decision with the patient whether they want the treatment or not.

In each of these contexts the importance of taking into account the consumers' views or perspectives was prescribed by professionals, managers and the government. In essence it is a **top-down prescriptive policy**. However, there is another context in which consumerism has been identified, and that is where consumerism in one form or another has emerged from initiatives taken by the population or segments of it (i.e. from the bottom up) – such as self-help groups and voluntary groups who represent clients unable to articulate fully their health needs and preferences.

These, then, are the general contexts in which consumer views and consumerism have been discussed in relation to health care. Using these different contexts as a background, the aim of this chapter is to outline and examine the consumers' perspective and the mechanisms and channels in the healthcare systems which are currently in place in the United Kingdom which reflect or are sensitive to consumers' interests.

THE RISE OF CONSUMERISM IN HEALTH CARE IN THE UK   The origins of the so-called consumer movement in health care in western society are difficult to trace, although it is claimed that there have over the last 50 years been changes in attitudes and expectations about health, medicine and health care. Williamson (1992) suggests that three different but interrelated elements contributed to the change in social consciousness that it is called consumerism in health care. These are:

♦ the creation of a climate of scepticism about medicine and medical care;

♦ the popularization of disturbing insights about professionals and institutions;

♦ the intense concern of small groups of patients or relatives.

Certainly there has been some discussion about the challenge to medicine from the articulate 'consumer'. It has been suggested (Elston 1991) that the 1980s witnessed not only the end of an era of optimism about scientific medicine but also the end of the era of the passive patient and the beginning of an era of active consumerism. At its simplest, it is argued that increased lay knowledge about medicine, declining deference to experts in society at large, changing attitudes of doctors and changing patterns of morbidity are modifying societal expectations about doctor–patient relationships in the direction of mutual participation. More specifically, there were three developments (Elston 1991).

♦ The first concerned the claims of interventionist medicines' ineffectiveness, of an epidemic iatrogenesis, of medicine's sapping of personal autonomy and the women's health movement's attacks on medicine. These all overtly challenged the professions' claim to be trusted with sole charge of the public's health.

♦ The second was the vigorous neo-liberal challenge to professional monopoly as inhibiting informed consumer choice. This emphasis on the discipline of the market and consumer power is echoed in the current reforms of the NHS – which will be discussed in detail later in the chapter.

♦ The third element of the challenge to medicine came from the dissatisfied patient: growing public concern about the professions' claim to effective self-discipline and medical malpractice in its widest sense. For example, the past decade appears to have seen a marked increase in overtly expressed complaints about the quality of medical care. As Allsop shows (1992), 1980s data sources indicate that members of the public were increasingly likely to lodge complaints about their health care. In 1977/78, 494 complaints were received by the Health Service Commissioner in the UK; by 1985/86 this had risen to 807. Similarly, service committee hearings involving GPs rose from 596 in 1977/78 to 1287 in 1985/86.

These are the arguments which have been put forward to explain the challenge from consumerism. However, there is more concrete evidence to show that 'consumerism' is growing. Allsop (1992) argues that self-help groups have become increasingly active. She shows, on the basis of selected data, that the public is making greater use of advisory services which are either wholly or partially concerned with health. For example, the number of branches of the National Childbirth Trust grew from 37 in 1971 to 353 in 1988. The family membership of the Leukaemia Care Society grew from

2000 in 1971 to 40 000 in 1988. There is also evidence to show that there has been an increase in the use of alternative therapies, and it is estimated that about 1.5 million patients consult alternative practitioners every year. However, it is difficult to judge whether this reflects scepticism about modern medicine or preference for better therapeutic relationships (Cant and Calnan 1991).

In summary, in this section some evidence has been presented which suggests that there has been an increase in 'consumerism' amongst the UK population as a whole or some segments of it. What has been the policy response?

GOVERNMENT POLICY AND CONSUMERISM

Government healthcare policy in the 1980s and 1990s has been characterized by its emphasis on market principles and managerialist ideals. Along with this has gone a great emphasis on consumer sovereignty, empowerment choice and the need for high-quality service with public responsiveness. These policies and their consequences will be discussed in more detail, although it must be remembered that there were mechanisms already in place to reflect the voice of the user before the very recent reforms.

In 1974, for example, the **Community Health Councils** were set up in every district to act as consumer watchdogs. Each CHC has between 18 and 24 members, half of whom are appointed by the local authority, one-third by local voluntary organizations and one-sixth by the regional health authority. CHCs have two major roles:

- ◆ The first is to keep under review the operation of the health services in the districts and to make recommendations for improvement. They have a right to visit NHS premises and to have access to information. They must be consulted on planning proposals and should publish an annual report.
- ◆ The second role is to provide information and advice to the public and particularly to those with special health needs. They also have a role in assisting complainants to bring their grievances to the attention of health authorities.

While CHCs have been useful in providing information to the public their powers are ill-defined and they have a low level of funding.

A wide variety of general and more specialized voluntary and self-help groups exist to provide information for the health service user and to act as pressure groups. Two of the most successful have been **AIMS** and **NAWCH**. Both were started in the early 1960s by mothers of young children. NAWCH believed that children's emotional development was best safeguarded, especially under the severe stress of being in hospital, by their parent's presence, and their basic standard for the psychosocial care of children in hospital was their unrestricted access to their parents (Williamson 1992).

One of the most interesting differences between NAWCH and AIMS was that, whereas NAWCH tended not to take up strictly clinical issues, AIMS felt no hesitation in studying and commenting on clinical

Pts/Citizens
challenge
The
Medical
Profession

matters. This was because AIMS defined pregnancy and childbirth as primarily socio-psychological events and not primarily medical-pathological ones, and thus every aspect of pregnancy and childbirth could come under AIMS scrutiny. The principle AIMS believed in was choice in childbirth – such as a woman's choice of whether to have the baby's father with her throughout labour and birth and for choice of place of birth. Since then AIMS has scrutinized each new obstetric technology as it has been introduced and has tried to protect a woman's right to refuse any intervention in the course of pregnancy or labour. These pressure groups in maternity and obstetric care are good examples of self-help groups trying to open up the channels to influence policy-making about health matters.

COMPLAINTS MECHANISMS

Procedures for handling complaints about the provision of services in the NHS fall into three main categories according to the type of grievance and the identity of the party against whom the complaint is made (Longley 1993).

Hospital complaints

Under Section 1 of the Hospital Complaints Procedure Act 1985, formal complaints about hospital services which do not involve the exercise of clinical judgement are referred to the relevant DHA, which has a nominated manager for dealing with them. Complaints which involve the exercise of clinical judgement are dealt with under separate procedures. The consultant concerned is required to examine the clinical aspects of the grievance. If the complainant is dissatisfied with the consultant's reply, the complaint can be referred in writing to the Regional Medical Officer or if necessary to the Independent Professional Review.

Family Health Service Authorities

Complaints about general practitioners are dealt with by the relevant FHSA with whom GPs are contracted to provide services. FHSAs can only formally investigate alleged breaches of terms of service which may include clinical judgement or other matters. The complaint must be made within 13 weeks of the course of action and is referred to a Medical Service Committee for investigation. A report is then made to the FHSA for a decision. Service Committees only consider specific allegations and incidents which might show a breach of contract. The Service Committee consists of three lay and three professional members in addition to the chairperson.

Complaints against general practitioners accused of professional misconduct, of being unfit to practice due to ill health or of criminal conduct are heard by the General Medical Council (GMC). The GMC can suspend a doctor's registration, strike the doctor off the register or reprimand the doctor concerned. More recently, the GMC agreed to investigate and lobby for a new professional offence of poor professional performance.

The Health Service Commissioner

The National Health Service Reorganisation Act 1973 established the post of **Health Service Ombudsman**. The Ombudsman can investigate a complaint brought by or on behalf of anyone who has suffered an 'injustice or hardship' due to a failure to provide a statutory service, or any type of maladministration. After each investigation the Health Service Commissioner issues a report. If the Commissioner is not satisfied with a health authority's response to the report, he or she can lay a report before the Secretary of State for Health and produce a special report for both houses of parliament.

The Health Service Commissioner dealt with only 124 cases between April 1991 and March 1992, although the number of complaints received has grown over the last decade. A case cannot usually be investigated by the Health Commissioner

- if the case involves clinical judgement;
- if the 'injustice or hardship' arises from lack of resources or national policy;
- if there is any alternative statutory mechanism the complainant might have used;
- if, in the opinion of the Commissioner, the complainant could reasonably have been expected to take formal legal action.

Overall, then, these are the complaints mechanisms that a dissatisfied consumer might follow. While there is evidence that formal complaints are increasing, these complaints mechanisms have been criticized for not being mutually exclusive, easily understandable and well-publicized. However, a recent review committee (Department of Health 1994) has recommended a simplified system with a common complaints mechanism: a recommendation which has been accepted by the UK government.

THE PATIENT'S CHARTER

Recent government policy has emphasized the importance of consumer choice and responsiveness, and this approach culminated in the **Patient's Charter** in 1991. However, before that, government policy documents concerned with primary care aimed to give patients better choice by providing them with more information about the services GPs offer, together with more competition amongst GPs and easier arrangements for changing doctors. The idea is that patients should be able to change their GP without first approaching their existing doctor and the FHSA. The idea of consumerism inherent in this proposal does not imply increased public participation in decision-making but is aimed at increasing 'individual' choice, as it is derived from a model of health care which suggests that its provision should be determined by a market economy.

The general principles of increased competition and consumer choice were also evident in the new reforms. However, this approach culminated in the Patient's Charter which emerged out of the Citizen's Charter (see Box 9.1).

Box 9.1
The Patient's Charter

Quality, choice, standards, and value are the charter's main themes. The Patient's Charter is believed to represent a fundamental shift towards consumer sovereignty. According to the Patient's Charter every citizen already has the following NHS rights:

◆ To receive health care on the basis of clinical need, regardless of ability to pay.
◆ To be registered with a GP.
◆ To receive emergency medical care at any time, through a GP or the emergency ambulance service and hospital accident and emergency departments.
◆ To be referred to a consultant, acceptable to the patient, when the GP thinks it necessary, and to be referred for a second opinion if the patient and the GP agree this is desirable.
◆ To be given a clear explanation of any treatment proposed, including any risks and any alternatives, before deciding whether to agree to the treatment.
◆ To have access to health records, and to know that those working for the NHS will, by law, keep their contents confidential.
◆ To choose whether or not to take part in medical research or medical student training.

In addition, from 1 April 1992 three new rights were introduced:

◆ To be given detailed information on local health services, including quality standards and maximum waiting times.
◆ To be guaranteed admission for virtually all treatments by a specific date, with no more than two years on a waiting list. Most patients will be admitted before this date. Currently 90% are admitted within a year.
◆ To have any complaint about NHS services – whoever provides them – investigated, and to receive a full and prompt written reply from the chief executive of the health authority or general manager of the hospital.

As yet, there is little evidence available to evaluate the impact of this initiative. However, there has been some criticism. For example, as Plamping and Delamothe state (1991):

'the extolling of choice, competition, and commitment to service suggests that the government equates citizens' rights with consumers' rights. To conflate the two, however, is to miss much of the point of citizenship. Active citizenship means giving citizens what they need to allow them to contribute fully to society. These needs include reasonable physical and mental health which cannot be adequately safeguarded by simply giving people rights as consumers. Consumers rights are contractual and have little meaning outside the market place where much caring takes place ... Consumers' rights are only that small subject of citizens' rights that relate to our experience in the market place'.

They conclude:

'The charter's commitment to quality is commendable, but without enfranchising those living in conditions of partial citizenship the charter is unlikely to contribute much to the health of the nation. Clearly stated individual rights might benefit the powerful and articulate, but they won't do much for those who lack the means to negotiate for their own health. Such a charter will not affect the lack of money or self confidence, nor will it affect the impact of chronic ill health or disability that reduces many peoples' ability to maintain a reasonable level of health'.

A key objective of the reformed NHS is to improve quality by making services more responsive to the needs and wishes of patients. The Patient's Charter is the cornerstone of the government's attempts to provide a quality service to patients. It is a compulsory subject for all purchasers and represents the minimum acceptable level of measurable quality performance demanded of all providers. **League tables** are to be published on five Charter topics:

- waiting times for assessment in A&E;
- waiting times in outpatient clinics;
- the cancelled operation standard;
- ambulance emergency response times;
- waiting times for admission in a number of specialties.

The idea is that the league tables should become an important part of the process of public accountability as the public has every right to know just how well the NHS is performing. Thus, in this context *empowerment* of patients is facilitated by information given. This approach to empowerment is a rather simplistic idea about obtaining autonomy and control (Saltmann 1994).

What has been the impact of the recent changes and the Patient's Charter on 'consumers'? One area where change has been beneficial is where patients were given access to their health records which was introduced in 1991. The evidence so far suggests that allowing patients to see their records as well as the correspondence between general practitioners and hospital doctors tends to improve communication and relationships between the three parties (Cartwright and Windsor 1992).

With regard to the limit on waiting list times, recent evidence (Cartwright and Windsor 1992) suggests that the Charter is targeting what may be a less important wait and doing it in an inefficient and inappropriate way. Patients seem to be more dissatisfied with the delay between referral by their general practitioner and being seen at an outpatient department and, to a lesser extent, the decision to put them on a waiting list.

Pts follow

Money

It is also unclear whether the changes or the new reforms will, on balance, increase or decrease patients' choices for hospitals. If patients end up 'following the money' rather than the money following the patients, they may have to travel further and their limited choices will be still more reduced. However, evidence seems to suggest that patient flows have contracted rather than expanded since the introduction of the internal market and there is little evidence as yet that money is following patients. District health authorities tend to negotiate 'block' contracts annually with providers and thus individual patient needs might be overlooked. These contracts probably are negotiated mainly according to the criteria of efficiency. General practitioners, particularly fund-holders, may be more sensitive to patient's individual needs, although early results suggest that budget holding has little influence on patient flow.

For example, Coulter and Bradlow (1993) compared the out-patient referral patterns in fundholding and non-fundholding practices before and after the implementation of the NHS reforms in April 1991. After the reforms there was no change in the proportion of referrals from the two groups of practices which crossed district boundaries. There was no evidence that fundholding was encouraging a shift from specialist to general practice or that budgetary pressures were affecting general practitioners' referral behaviour, such as to private clinics. However, one context where general practitioners have more flexibility and can tailor their referrals to individual needs is extracontractual referrals, and that is where money might follow patients.

Alternatively ✳

CHOICE AND HEALTH CARE

For some the term 'consumer' could be replaced by 'patient' or 'user'. For others, the notion of consumer has been linked with consumer sovereignty and the market economy. Unlike consumers of other commodities, those seeking medical care are constrained by their lack of knowledge of the choices available and are dependent on professional expertise, especially in life-threatening situations. Certainly, one aspect which is particularly associated with health and health care is *uncertainty*. The intrinsically unequal nature of the relationship between provider and consumers means that consumers are not in a position to shop around for the best buy and make informed choices – as those who advocate a business model of health care assume. Moreover, the distinction between the consumer and the producer of health care is not as clear-cut as some might think, as ordinary people are also responsible for producing good health and preventing illness.

Government policy, as was shown earlier, has emphasized the need to make more choices available to consumers. However, choice in health care is not as easy as in other economic markets specifically because health care has unique characteristics. Thus, with the fundholding initiative a patient is still dependent on the GP purchasing on their behalf. Any choice is exercised by the GP who decides where to place contracts. In this respect patients of a fundholder may have extended choice in that their GP is able to make extracontractual referrals should the need arise.

There are a number of other areas where government policies have attempted to extend choice. One is in choosing a GP, and the reforms have sought to encourage patients to act as consumers and shop around for their health care. However, several authors (e.g. Leavy *et al.*, 1989) are sceptical of this happening – they question patients' motivation to act as consumers and their enthusiasm for shopping around. They argue that most people change their doctor only when circumstances force them to do so, either because they have moved or because their general practitioner has moved, retired or died. The nature of peoples' need for GP services and the circumstances in which they arise may militate against motivating people to embark on a search for a new doctor. Many peoples' contact with their GP is minimal and spasmodic – perhaps once a year for a prescription – so it may seem a waste of time to think of alternatives. If an urgent condition does arise then it would preclude the possibility of shopping around. For those with chronic conditions, a relationship of trust and confidence may have been built up during the course of an illness which provides a powerful incentive to stay put.

Similarly, the question of choice with regard to exit from the public sector into the private sector is more complicated than it appears. Survey evidence (Calnan *et al.*, 1993) has consistently shown general loyalty and support for the NHS. The vast majority believe that the government should have a responsibility for the provision of health care and there has been an increase in those who believe the state should spend more on the health services. However, there has been an increase in dissatisfaction with the NHS at least between 1983 and 1990, and the major source of dissatisfaction was with attending hospital as an outpatient, and to a lesser extent, being in hospital as an inpatient. Concern about hospital services focused mainly on the hospital waiting list for a non-emergency operation and the waiting time before getting an appointment with a hospital consultant. This increase in dissatisfaction with hospital care appears to coincide with the growth in the proportion of the population covered by *private health insurance*, and the vast majority of people who use private health care acute services now have private insurance coverage. By 1981 the percentage insured was 7%, by 1989 it had peaked at 13%, although more recently this percentage has begun to fall. However, the survey evidence which suggests that dissatisfaction with the NHS is a major reason for subscribing to private health insurance is misleading, and such dissatisfaction does not neces-

*Consumer
Sovereignty* (handwritten annotation)

sarily affect subscribers' broad principles about the organization and funding of the healthcare system. People appear to hold private health insurance for a number of reasons (Calnan *et al.* 1993), the major one being that they are offered it as a 'perk' by an employer.

Does the use of private health insurance increase 'consumer choice'? The evidence (Calnan *et al.* 1993) suggests that choice is extended only slightly. Certainly, those who had experienced private health care stressed the quality of the facilities and the individualized nature of care and timing of visit; but there was little evidence of shopping around between the private and public sectors. Also, subscribers had limited knowledge of their insurance policy and the costs of treatment and felt they lacked the competence to evaluate the skills of different consultants in order to make an informed choice. Rather than shopping around for the best deal, they depended on their GP to decide whether they should go privately and if so which consultant they should see. Thus, the notion of consumer sovereignty in this context at least was problematic and individuals did not feel more empowered or more knowledgeable.

QUALITY AND THE CONSUMER

Much of the discussion so far has focused on the issue of time and the value patients put on reducing delays in access to health care. Certainly, the rationing of time appears to be an issue which is discussed in the context of most forms of healthcare systems, although it is a particular problem associated with systems such as the NHS. The issue of time is an important issue also in the context of certain special services. For example, at the hospital casualty or accident and emergency departments the majority of patients are 'walk in' patients who know what is wrong with them and require effective treatment as quickly as possible. However, there are other aspects of quality of care which consumers perceive as important.

One aspect which is perceived to be important irrespective of the type of service provided or the setting in which it is provided is the quality of the professional–patient relationships (see Box 9.2).

The nature and quality of the doctor–patient relationship is of particular importance in general practice and there was some concern that the changes in the new GP contract in 1990 would have a detrimental effect on it – in that the changes might have accorded a more formal and bureaucratic role to the GP with less time in the consultation. The results of a recent study comparing consumer perceptions before (in 1988) and after (1991) the new GP contract was implemented (Calnan *et al.* 1994) showed that these fears were unfounded. Overall satisfaction with the general practitioner was broadly similar in 1988 and 1991 and there was little change in concerns about time restriction. Nevertheless, the

Box 9.2
Predictors of consumer
satisfaction – an
example

Williams and Calnan (1991) examined the extent to which there is convergence or divergence in assessing the criteria of consumer satisfaction across general practice, dental and hospital care settings. Their findings showed clearly that issues concerning professional competence, together with the nature and quality of the patient–professional relationship, were consistently the most important predictors of overall consumer satisfaction with general practice, dental and hospital care. Some typical comments were:

'I never feel my GP has enough time for me and therefore often end up telling him only half the reason why I came'.

'I feel very much at ease with [my dentist] because he always explains what is necessary to be done'.

'I was dissatisfied [in hospital] because basically there was no personal care given and the doctors were unfriendly and they didn't bother to try and treat my needs and worries separately'.

*factors
for
liking
GPs*

question of *quality of time* in the consultation still remains a difficult issue. The importance for the patient of the doctor–patient relationship in general practice was also clearly shown in this study. Box 9.3 shows that the strongest influences of overall satisfaction with general practice were whether the doctor was understanding, had good medical skills, was good at explaining things and was liked as a person. Thus, the findings once again demonstrate the continued importance of the more diffuse social and psychological aspects of primary care to the consumer.

In other settings there are also specific aspects which patients emphasize. For example, for hospital inpatient services (Fitzpatrick 1984) rigid timetables, poor quality of meals and a lack of privacy are sources of complaints. In breast cancer screening services (Vaile *et al.* 1993) concern with the pain and discomfort of the mammogram and delay in receiving results were the important sources of dissatisfaction.

In areas such as general practice and breast screening services overall consumer satisfaction levels are high – indicating that quality is high. In a recent study of general practice (Calnan *et al.* 1994), 97% were satisfied specifically with their general practitioner and 86% thought their primary care rather than just their GP to be good or very good. Questions about specific aspects of primary care also showed generally high level of satisfaction. For example, 85% of respondents were satisfied with the access they had to their GPs, although a lower level of satisfaction was found with their practice's preventive care. In the case of breast screening (Vaile *et al.* 1993) a recent study of attenders in three districts

Box 9.3
Ranked summary of
zero correlations
between various
aspects of health care
and overall satisfaction
with GP

Question	Overall satisfaction with GP (Spearman's rho)
Doctor generally understanding	0.68 ($p < 0.01$)
Doctor has good medical skills	0.62 ($p < 0.0001$)
Doctor good at explaining things	0.61 ($p < 0.0001$)
Like GP as a person	0.60 ($p < 0.0001$)
Satisfied with out-of-hours care	0.58 ($p < 0.0001$)
Overall satisfaction with access	0.52 ($p < 0.0001$)
Examines thoroughly	0.50 ($p < 0.0001$)
GP gives enough information	0.50 ($p < 0.0001$)
GP spends enough time in consultation	0.48 ($p < 0.0001$)
Satisfaction with family planning advice	0.48 ($p < 0.001$)
GP spent enough time in consultation	0.39 ($p < 0.0001$)
Well equipped surgery	0.34 ($p < 0.001$)
Helpful receptionist	0.33 ($p < 0.001$)
Usefulness of practice leaflet	0.33 ($p < 0.001$)
GP good at referrals to other agencies	0.31 ($p < 0.0001$)
Waiting time too long	0.28 ($p < 0.001$)
Basic socio-demographic parameters	
Age	-0.17 ($p < 0.0001$)
Education	0.10 ($p < 0.0001$)
Health over last 12 months	-0.06 (not significant)
Social class	0.02 (not significant)

showed satisfaction averaged 4.5 on our five-point scale and 95% of the combined sample said they would return when invited in three years' time.

In other areas or settings dissatisfaction is higher. As was mentioned earlier, hospital services occasion more dissatisfaction than general practitioner services. Concern about hospital services focuses mainly on the hospital waiting list for a non-emergency operation and the waiting time before getting an appointment with a hospital consultant. In the 1990 Social Attitudes Survey (Calnan et al. 1993), 83% and 82%, respectively, said these areas were in need of a lot or some improvement. However, in other areas such as services for people with disabilities and those who are chronically sick, levels of satisfaction are lower. For example, in a study of patients' evaluation of the Artificial Limb Service (Limb et al. 1993) based on a sample of above-knee amputees ($N = 110$), 64% expressed dissatisfaction with the service and the major causes of concern were in the areas of communication, comfort and choice. Users were particularly dissatisfied with the fitting of the limbs and lack of counselling and support. Certainly, this seems to indicate that this type of service is of low quality – although in this setting sufferers, because of their regular visits to health care about the same problem and having to live with the problem, become expert and well-informed themselves and are thus able to be more critical of professional practice. The continuity of contact makes the effectiveness or ineffectiveness of care more visible to the consumer.

Satisfaction varies not only with the type of service provided but also with the characteristics of the patient population being served. For example, among those who have had recent treatment, satisfaction levels tend to be higher than with those who have not recently used the specific service. Also, of the socio-demographic characteristics of the population age is the most important influence and satisfaction seems to increase with age. This finding may reflect real differences in the actual experience of health care; or it may reflect lower *expectations* of the older generation, or more *realistic* expectations in that they experienced the health service pre-NHS or do not expect too much of modern medicine and accept its limitations. Alternatively, the older generation may have a greater degree of deference and respect for the medical profession as a whole, although this may be 'strategic' in that they use the professional medical care more often than their younger counterparts.

SUMMARY

This chapter has examined the healthcare system from the perspective of the patient, or what is now termed the consumer. It has outlined why patients' or consumers' perspectives should be taken into account and shown how government policy has changed particularly in the last few years. Certainly, the ideology has shifted away from a public participation model where there are specific mechanisms and structures set up to channel the public views into the policy decision-making, towards an approach which emphasizes the principles of the market economy and consumer sovereignty where the focus is on tailoring services to consumer demand and enabling choice.

There is no evidence that consumers have been given any power in the NHS to participate in decision-making. The Community Health Councils are a part of the consultation machinery although there is no obligation to act on their views. More recent approaches put an emphasis on information-giving, although how far the views of the public are fed back or taken on board by managers is difficult to tell. Certainly, active participation is not encouraged, and the complaints mechanisms are set up to protect consumer rights rather than to promote them. Thus, since the inception of the NHS, while there is little evidence of 'Exit', there is also little evidence that the voice of the consumer has had a powerful influence on decision-making and recent policy has done little to change this. Empowerment and effective citizen participation requires managers to do more than provide crude information about waiting times and commission surveys of the public's views. It requires the setting up of structures and mechanisms where the public or their selected representatives have at least the negotiating power to *influence* decisions (Saltmann 1994).

FURTHER READING

◆ Journals: These issues are covered in journals such as *Sociology of Health and Illness* and *Social Science and Medicine*.

◆ Calnan, M., Cant, S. and Gabe, J. (1993), *Going Private: Why People Pay for their Care*. Open University Press, Buckingham.

◆ Gabe, J., Calnan, M. and Bury, M. (Eds) (1991), *Sociology of the Health Service*, Routledge, London.

◆ Williamson, C. (1992), *Whose Standards? Consumer and Professional Standards in Health Care*. Open University Press, Buckingham.

REFERENCES

Allsop, J. (1992), The voice of the user in health care. In: Beck, E., Lonsdale, S., Newman, S. and Patterson, D. (Eds), *In the Best of Health*. London: Chapman & Hall.

Calnan, M., Cant, S. and Gabe, J. (1993), *Going Private: Why People Pay for their Care*. Buckingham: Open University Press.

Calnan, M., Coyle, J. and Williams, S. (1994), Changing perceptions of general practitioner care, *European Journal of Public Health*, 4:108–14.

Cant, S. and Calnan, M. (1991), On the margins of the medical market place, *Sociology of Health and Illness*, 13(1):39–57.

Cartwright, A. and Windsor, J. (1992), *Outpatients and Their Doctors*. London: HMSO.

Coulter, A. and Bradlow, J. (1993), Effect of NHS reforms on general practitioners' referral patterns, *BMJ*, 306:433–7.

Department of Health (1994), *Being Heard. The Report of a Review Committee on NHS Complaints Procedure*. London: Department of Health.

Elston, M. (1991), The politics of professional power. In: Gabe, J., Calnan, M. and Bury, M. (Eds), *Sociology of the Health Service*. London: Routledge.

Fitzpatrick, R. (1984), Satisfaction with health care. In: Fitzpatrick, R., Hinton, J., Newman, S., Scambler, G. and Thompson, J. (Eds), *The Experience of Illness*. London: Tavistock.

Leavy, R., Wilkin, D. and Metcalfe, D.H.M. (1989), Consumerism and general practice, *BMJ*, 298:737–9.

Limb, M., Limb, J. and Calnan, M. (1993), Reach for the sky, *Health Service Journal*, 103:26–8.

Longley, D. (1993), *Public Law and Health Service Accountability*. Buckingham: Open University Press.

Plamping, O. and Delamothe, A. (1991), The Citizens' Charter and the NHS, *BMJ*, 303:203.

Saltmann, R.B. (1994), Patient choice and patient empowerment in Northern European health systems: A conceptual framework. *International Journal of Health Services*, 24(2):201–29.

Vaile, M., Calnan, M., Rutter, D. and Wall, B. (1993), Uptake and response to breast cancer screening services in three areas, *Public Health Medicine*, 15(1):37–45.

Williams, S. J. and Calnan, M. (1991), Convergence and divergence: assessing criteria of consumer satisfaction across general practice, dental and hospital care settings, *Social Science and Medicine*, 33(6):707–16.

Williamson, C. (1992), *Whose Standards? Consumer and Professional Standards in Health Care*. Buckingham: Open University Press.

THE MANAGEMENT AGENDA FOR SENIOR CLINICIANS

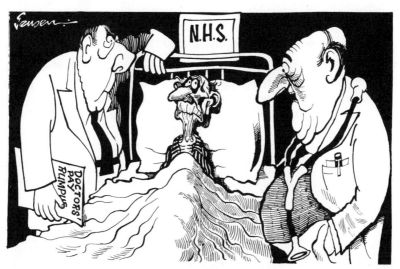

"You'll have to have another transfusion – from you to us, that is."

(First published in the *Sunday Telegraph*, 7 June 1970)

It is inconceivable that clinicians can avoid being partners in the management of the institutions in which they work.

As custodians of the technology of health care, clinical managers must ensure that the resources they require are available at the correct time and in the right quantities. They must be sure that health services do not stop at the level of providing effective procedures but that those procedures are delivered in the form of effective services which meet the needs of relevant populations. To do so in the 'new NHS' requires a working knowledge of the pattern and mechanisms by which services are delivered and the skills to use management processes such as planning, budgeting, control, and quality management in the interests of patients and the development of services.

This volume has not been able to cover issues in the depth which the subject requires or to cover all changes in a dynamic field. Further volumes have been commissioned which cover key issues such as:

♦ contracting for Services;
♦ achieving Value for Money;
♦ the Role of the Clinical Director; and
♦ management in General Practice.

Each of the chapters in this book can be seen as a broad introduction to the area and the bibliographies should provide a strong starting point for more detailed analysis.

We conclude the volume by identifying some of the main issues for clinical managers which arise throughout this volume. The editors are clear that these will form an important part of the management agenda for senior clinicians for some years to come.

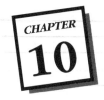

CHAPTER

10

LOOKING FORWARDS

David A. Perkins

INTRODUCTION

In the introduction to this volume it was suggested that effective management of a complex organization required: objectives that are long-term, simple and agreed; a profound understanding of the competitive environment; and an objective appraisal of resources. While various stakeholders within the NHS are very clear about their objectives, and indeed various Ministers of Health have attempted to restate those objectives since the passing of the NHS Act in 1946, it would be hard to argue that the NHS or its component institutions share a clear and coherent set of objectives.

For much of the time this is not an important impediment to the provision of services to patients, but it becomes problematic when the inherent conflicts over resources become explicit. Indeed many of the new trusts and purchaser organizations have attempted to spell out their objectives in more detail to focus the management process. Much of this volume has concerned the specific environment in which health services operate and the management of the resources and capabilities with which care is delivered. This chapter starts by commenting on the broad context for health care and gradually focuses to look at some of the issues as they affect clinical and departmental management. In no way is this a substitute for reading the contributions and the review is by no means exhaustive.

THE CONTEXT FOR HEALTH CARE

Unfortunately the context in which the NHS operates is not consistent and there is little evidence that it will become so. Talk of a 'level playing field' seems to belong to the language of political rhetoric rather than practical experience. Some aspects of this environment are amenable to local or even individual action while others are fixed and perhaps unknowable. Important issues will be drawn from the contributions in this volume raising some of the key challenges for the NHS and its clinicians.

Several contributors point to the epidemiological and demographic contexts and their impact on services. These phenomena consist of many processes that are broadly predictable and others that are characterized by their scale and unpredictability. The ageing population with its high levels of dependency is not news. This trend has been apparent for a number of years yet the service responses from health and social service agencies are less than adequate. Combined with a decade of weak economic performance, high unemployment and changes in family structure and values, the impact of this trend has been to vastly increase the demands placed upon organizations who have little idea how it might be met. In contrast, the development of AIDS and services to meet it has been unpredictable. From the clinical research findings of the early 1980s to government health promotion activities and additional ring-fenced funding for each locality, we have moved to a position where funding for AIDS services is to be seen as part of the normal resources available to purchasers. An unpredictable infectious disease has become a top priority for a limited period and is now in process of becoming normalized – one of the many demands to be considered by purchasers and placed in priority order.

The national economic performance has many effects on the NHS but it principally impacts through the levels and priorities attributed to it in decisions about public expenditure and in the decisions made by individuals and corporations about the private purchase and provision of health care. Social factors which impact on demand for services include:

♦ the extent to which the population develops healthy diets and exercise patterns;
♦ the social acceptability or otherwise of smoking and;
♦ what is sometimes euphemistically referred to as 'the caring capacity of the community'.

These components of the demand system are neither independent nor isolated – which adds to their complexity, both in terms of their effects and their impact but also in their timing. For instance, the attempt to identify targets in *The Health of the Nation* implies that we have some understanding of the social processes involved in the trends for teenage pregnancies or for drug abuse and that we might be able to influence such trends for the good within an agreed timescale.

THE BEHAVIOUR OF GOVERNMENT

Governments of all persuasions respond to the various demands by attempting to increase the effectiveness of public and social institutions or occasionally by finding an appropriate scapegoat. Since complex problems usually have equally complex causes, we find a growing recognition that important problems require action by several agencies in concert and that isolated action is often counterproductive. Thus *Health of the Nation* introduces the jargon of 'healthy alliances', and the late Sir Roy Griffiths in his second report insisted that health, social service, and voluntary agencies should work together with carers to improve the lot of those in need of community care (DoH 1990; Griffiths 1988). The demands made of hard-pressed agencies for complex joint planning are considerable, even where there is the incentive of special additional funds for the purpose. The fear of accepting funds, developing new services, and being left 'holding the baby' if those funds are no longer available has created a sense of caution among provider organizations. More simply, the complexity of joint care agreements, often developed through case conferences, can be significant for individual patients without trying to develop joint services for communities.

The government is continually subject to the criticism that its services do not meet legitimate needs and therefore a response which questions the effectiveness and efficiency of its services is not surprising. The development of the National Audit Office, the Audit Commission, and other bodies charged with increasing the efficiency of services, has resulted in many reports but rather fewer control systems to influence the patterns of management and resource use. This may, of course, be only a matter of time since the services which it seeks to influence are complicated and the basic underlying technology of care is located in the minds of clinicians and other practitioners. For instance, the development of a national research and development capacity for the NHS is based on the principle that effective treatments and services can be distinguished from ineffective ones and that expenditure can be focused on proven treatments and services. There are, however, a number of commentators who point to the remarkable resilience of ineffective treatments, to iatrogenesis and cross-infection in hospitals, which suggests that the impact of such R&D strategies might not be straightforward (Illich 1977).

In response to social developments, and possibly as a means of covering a perceived gap between the available resources and those which consumers and providers would like, the government has introduced the Charter movement which provides mechanisms for compensating individuals inconvenienced by inefficient state agencies. These developments might be interpreted as visible actions designed to ward off criticism and garner public support; but on the other hand they might be real attempts to deal with difficult problems. It is not immediately clear that the Citizen's Charter cuts much ice in a busy, oversubscribed outpatient clinic. Whether we can expect further developments, more robust targets and control, and more serious sanctions remains to be seen. It may be OK to penalize British Rail for late trains but not to sanction the overworked hospital for late appointments. This does, of course, assume that the majority of outpatient appointments are necessary or indeed useful to the patient – but this points to fundamental questions about the pattern of care which we shall return to later.

Governments are always likely to undertake highly visible actions to deal with issues of symbolic or real importance particularly if they can be achieved at minimal cost. For example, the government has announced £4.4 million in new funds to set up secure units for the severely mentally ill to ward off criticisms from an enquiry by the Mental Health Foundation that the community-based services do not meet the needs of this group (Brindle 1994).

THE MARKET

A number of contributors to this volume point out that a mechanism has been set in place and it is not clear what the outcomes will be. The structure of the market assumes that the prime purchasing influences are 'bottom-up', albeit with some attention paid to government priorities and national programmes. This represents the abandonment of the **normative** principle that there are standards for the levels of provision which ought to be achieved, whether expressed in terms of the number of beds or the number of procedures or treatments carried out per head of a target population. Rather the market assumes that needs are identified and appropriate services are secured by the contractor despite the fact that the specialist medical skills are largely confined to the provider trusts.

This situation enables the trust and its staff to exercise more influence in the contracting process than might be expected, but it does require that clinicians are aware of the contracting process and are prepared to make an effective case for their services. Many trusts have identified this activity as 'marketing' and have appointed specialist managers, but it may be more effective if clinicians are aware of the possibilities within the contracting process since they have the specialist knowledge with which to convince sceptical purchasers.

The purchasers

The purchaser has the option of buying services from providers in the public or private sectors. While the majority of purchasing, especially for sophisticated procedures, will be from NHS trusts, some care will be bought from the private sector which appears to have excess capacity at the moment. Although such contracts for services or extracontractual referrals appear to be the exception rather than the rule, it is important to be aware of the reasons for such purchases. Frequently the private sector is seen to offer a flexibility not available in conventional services, and while this cannot always be mirrored in public hospitals, it is not often, apart from loss-leaders, that the private sector can compete on price.

Relationships between purchasers and providers are critical since the possibility of switching from one provider to another is ever-present. In those specialist areas that depend on individual referrals, such as some areas of psychiatry, each referral may constitute a separate decision. Likewise some fundholding practices may make significant referrals and be sufficiently flexible to change providers depending on their view of the particular strengths offered by a particular service, or indeed individual consultant. It follows that many heads of service are going to want to meet a wide range of purchasers on a regular basis to promote their own department or institution. Where the relationships between purchasers and providers become adversarial rather than cooperative it is likely that both sides will lose out and the service will suffer.

As indicated above, the purchasing of complex services will cause difficulties for purchaser and provider. While some needs may be standardized using a simple protocol, others will require the services of a number of specialties combined in a particular pattern or working together in tandem. Indeed some patients who present with simple diagnoses will turn out, following investigation, to require more sophisticated treatments and care programmes.

It should not be forgotten that there will need to be contracts, or at least service-level agreements, between departments which provide direct services to patients and those which provide support services such as imaging and pathology. The efficient management of departments may require complex discharge arrangements to ensure that patients can receive appropriate levels of social care to facilitate discharge and rehabilitation.

While the purchasing activity has focused on short-term issues, in particular the negotiation of contracts, it has also to take account of long-term issues. The continued provision of services may require capital developments which are likely to be as difficult as ever to secure. The purchasing of education and training is largely the responsibility of the employer, but the size of trusts makes it likely that they will need to act in consortia with other trusts to maintain economic training numbers and to even out the fluctuations of demand patterns so that the provider institutions, largely in higher and further education, are willing to invest in appropriate and relevant programmes of basic and more advanced training.

Research will be purchased by a variety of charities, commercial organizations, research councils, and government departments and it is likely that market principles will prevail. Trusts will want to be clear that all costs are met and that there is an appropriate contribution to the host organization, while purchasers will want to be clear that their investment is managed appropriately. The traditional placing of research contracts in teaching and postgraduate institutions is likely to become more competitive, with large trusts becoming more professional in their handling of the research process.

THE PROVIDER SYSTEM

The separation of providers though the creation of semi-independent trusts is bound to have an impact on the provision of a seamless service. Since the efficiency of the service depends on patients receiving an appropriate level of care to meet their needs, the separation of providers must permit competition and cooperation.

Separate providers may need to create service-level agreements to ensure the availability of services for which they are not equipped, which are oversubscribed, or which are not economic for two trusts to provide. It is clear from the history of organizational strategies that where two organizations attempt to compete head-to-head they may both be damaged.

A further feature of the provider system that is unresolved is the question of successful and unsuccessful providers. If one trust is able to reduce the unit cost of its services while maintaining acceptable quality it is likely to obtain more contracts and grow. It may take over the management of services provided by another trust, thus increasing its income at the expense of its competitors. What is to become of the less successful trust? A reduction in income requires a consequent reduction in costs and either a scaling down of activities or a dramatic increase in efficiency. The options would appear to include a change in focus of the trust through some form of specialization or change in its core identity, a change in management, the merger with a more successful trust, or indeed closure if there is excess capacity at a neighbouring provider and there is no overriding political objection.

Provider management
It can be seen from the above that the successful provider institution will require a combination of systems, skills, and commitment if it is to operate successfully in the market. Relevant and timely information and the systems for handling it cannot be developed overnight and the skills of interpretation may take longer. In the past clinicians have shown little faith in the quality of management information and therefore such information as has been available has been put to limited use. Nonetheless such information is vital and much of it is built upon the activity information provided by clinicians – which is seldom understood by those responsible for processing that information. It follows that if the management of trusts is built on such information systems it is in the interests of clinicians to ensure that it is as accurate as possible. But the accuracy of information only forms a base since from it must stem active management of the activities concerned.

While it is attractive to contemplate the standardization of information systems throughout the NHS, the unfortunate experiences of the London Stock Exchange, Wessex Regional Health Authority, and the Department of Social Security in their attempts to devise comprehensive computer information systems should prove salutary. Such systems may be developed but perhaps we should not wait too eagerly nor trust in their promises.

'SAFE IN OUR HANDS'
While she was Prime Minister, Margaret Thatcher announced, in a phrase that has been repeated many times, that the NHS is 'safe in our hands'. What then of the future? The market mechanism cannot

be expected to ensure that the NHS remains as an equitable – or even as an efficient – provider of health services. That is down to the efforts of the clinicians and managers who plan and manage the service taking care to ensure that the short-term crises do not endanger the long-term future of health services in the UK.

REFERENCES

Brindle, D. (1994), £4.4 million for secure units for the mentally ill, *Guardian*, 8 Sept., p. 4.

Department of Health (1990), *The Health of the Nation: A Strategy for Health in England*. London: HMSO.

Griffiths, R. (1988), *Community Care: Agenda for Action*. London: HMSO.

Illich, I. (1977), *Disabling Professions*. London: Marion Boyars.

McKeown, T. (1976), *The Role of Medicine*. London: Nuffield Provincial Hospitals Trust.

GLOSSARY

Absorption Costing   An approach to determining the unit cost of products under which each unit of the product is charged with its full share of fixed costs. It is sometimes referred to as full costing.

AIMS   Association for the Improvement of Maternity Services.

Audit Commission   Independent public body charged with the audit of services provided by health services and local government.

Block Contracts   A form of contract which specifies a given number of treatments to be provided at an average price.

Budget   A formal quantified statement (normally expressed in financial terms) of a plan of action.

Budget Variance   The difference between the amount contained in a budget and the corresponding actual cost or revenue.

Capital funding   The funding for buildings and equipment which have a significant life expectancy, usually more than a calendar year.

Cash Flow   The actual cash receipts and payments of an enterprise for a particular accounting period.

Cash Limits   The determination of a fixed cash sum from which services must be provided.

Cash Planning   The planning of services within a fixed cash sum.

Community Care Plans   Plans for providing care in the community which frequently involve the cooperation of statutory and voluntary agencies.

Compulsory Competitive Tendering (CCT)   A government policy requiring public services to produce clear specifications of the services they provide and to seek tenders to provide these services from the private sector with the intention of ensuring high standards of efficiency and management practice.

Controllable Cost   A cost that can be directly controlled at a given level of management.

Cost and Volume Contracts   A more sophisticated form of contract which triggers changes in price to reflect changes in costs at different volumes of service.

Cost Centre   A responsibility centre within an enterprise, the performance of which is assessed in terms of the service it provides and the costs that it incurs in providing that service.

Costs by Behaviour A form of costing which examines whether costs are fixed regardless of volume, vary directly with volume or rise in a step-wise fashion.

Costs by Service A form of cost allocation which attributes cost to the particular services in which they are incurred.

Dawson Report A government report of a committee chaired by Lord Dawson of Penn published in 1920 which addressed the most appropriate structure of hospital and related services.

Dependency Models Statistical models which attempt to calculate the needs, usually for nursing care, of patients with different types and severity of clinical conditions thus allowing a calculation of how many care staff of what grades and experience are required at a particular time.

Depreciation The process of allocating the net cost (original acquisition cost minus estimated scrap value) of a long lived asset over its estimated life.

Direct Cost A cost which is specifically and measurably identified with a particular activity within an enterprise. Such costs are sometimes referred to as separable costs.

District Health Authority (DHA) An authority covering one or more local government areas which is responsible for assessing health needs and ensuring that they are provided. This is now achieved by purchasing care from Provider Units.

Efficiency Index An index used to compare the relative efficiency of services within the NHS and of the NHS itself in comparable time periods.

Efficiency Scrutinies Studies which are undertaken to assess the efficiency of clinical or support services which often give advice on best practice as a means of improving management.

Executive Agencies New organization forms developed as a means of simplifying responsibilities for services which were frequently the responsibility of departments of the Civil Service or Ministries of State.

External Financing Limits The limits imposed by central government on the annual use of external finance by public sector organizations.

Family Health Services Authority (FHSA) The authority responsible for managing the contracts of general practitioners, dentists, pharmacists and opticians. Usually, but not always, covers the same area as a DHA.

Financial Management Initiative A government initiative to improve the management of public funds in government departments with the objective of improving value for money and accountability.

Fixed Capital Items such as the premises or equipment.

Functional Accounting Accounting systems organized around the particular functions of an organization such as estate management, hotel services, clinical services etc.

General Practitioner A doctor of first contact. After qualification a general practitioner has to spend three years in further training before he or she can be admitted as a Principal in general practice. At least one year must be as a trainee in general practice. From 1996 there will be an assessment of this training, but many potential general practitioners currently take the Membership Examination of the Royal College of General Practitioners.

GP Fundholder A GP practice which holds a budget for services that can be purchased from hospitals and other providers of health and social care on behalf of patients.

Health Service Ombudsman The officer who is the final arbiter in the complaints procedure before the courts. Until recently, excluded from complaints about clinical service and decision: the remit is to be extended to include this area as well.

Incremental Scrutinies Examinations which relate to marginal changes or developments in a service or other activity as opposed to complete reviews of the whole activity.

Indirect Cost See Overhead costs.

Individual Performance Appraisal A system for the assessment of an individual's performance in their job and the examination of their potential for development and appropriate forms of training and other support to exploit this potential.

Internal Market The NHS 'market' which resulted from the separation of those who plan and purchase local services and those who provide those services through the medium of a contract or service agreement.

Joint Commissioning/Joint Purchasing Where services are purchased by more than one agency, frequently health authorities and social service departments.

Local Medical Committees (LMCs) A committee composed of local GPs and other independent practitioners through which they attempt to influence purchasers and defend their own interests.

Marginal Cost The increase in total costs associated with an increase in activity levels (usually of one unit).

Market Testing Initiative See CCT. This is where a public service produces a specification of its services and seeks tenders from other organizations to see if those services could be provided more efficiently or effectively.

Medical Audit Advisory Groups (MAAGs) Committees set up to advise on the efficacy of medical audit procedures in provider settings.

Mental Illness Specific Grant Central Government grant to Local Authorities tied to services for the mentally ill.

Merrison Commission The Royal Commission on the NHS which reported in 1979.

NHS Management Executive   The 'management board' and its officers which are responsible to the Secretary of State for the NHS and its management.

National Audit Office   The body responsible for the audit of those services provided by government departments and executive agencies.

NAWCH   National Association for Women and Children in Hospitals.

Near Patient Testing   The use of pathological tests within the surgery as opposed to sending specimens to a laboratory for analysis. This allows rapid results and facilitates quick action but may not be cost effective.

New Public Management   A new approach to public management which builds heavily on private sector approaches to managing organizations.

Normative Views   Statements which suggest a normal or appropriate level, standard, or approach to a particular issue. For instance, there should be x beds per 10 000 population.

Opportunity Cost   An economic concept which regards the costs of utilizing a resource as the benefit foregone by not using it in its best alternative use.

Overhead Costs   The costs which are not directly associated with a particular activity. These are sometimes referred to as indirect costs.

Patient Participation Groups   Groups of patients who contribute their views to the running and development of services, often found in general practice settings.

Patient Satisfaction Surveys   Surveys to assess the level of patient satisfaction with health services.

Performance Related Pay   A system of pay in which there is a component linked to the performance of the individual in the previous year.

Pluralism   An approach which recognizes and permits a range of different interests to influence the policy process and the decisions which are made.

Public Sector Borrowing Requirements (PSBR)   The amount of money which the government borrows to balance its annual income and expenditure.

Resource Allocation Working Party (RAWP)   A working party and then a formula which was used in the 1980s to redistribute funds from health services in the over-provided south to the under-provided north on the grounds of a definition of need.

Semi-Variable Costs   Costs which have both a fixed and variable element.

Staff Satisfaction Surveys   Surveys to assess the levels of staff satisfaction within their place of work which is often seen to be related to motivation.

Subjective Accounting   The traditional NHS form of accounting for expenditure in which reports allocated expenditure to the input headings e.g. staff, utilities, drugs, etc.

Tomlinson Report   The report of a committee set up to review the pattern of healthcare services in London and make recommendations.

Total Quality Management   An approach to quality management originating in the private sector which claims to be comprehensive.

Transaction Costs   The costs incurred in purchasing a service that are additional to the cost of the service provided. Thus the administrative costs of an extracontractual referral are transaction costs and may be significant if there are many ECRs.

Unit Cost   The total (full) cost of producing one unit of a good or service.

Variable Costs   Costs where the total amount varies as the level of activity changes.

Whitley Council   A system of negotiation in which representatives of staff and management negotiated over pay and conditions in the NHS: it was often found to be bulky and bureaucratic.

Zero-Based Budgeting   A system of budgeting originally developed in the USA for non-trading organizations. Its approach is bottom-up and involves the ranking of the contribution that differing activities make to the achievement of organizational objectives in cost/benefit terms.

INDEX

Note: terms explained in the Glossary are indicated by **bold page numbers**; text in Boxes, Figures and Tables, by *italic page numbers*. Index entries are arranged in letter-by-letter order (ignoring spaces).